W9-AAP-624

Advance Praise for *30 Days to a More Powerful Memory*

"Anyone can train their memory to be "fitter and stronger," and this book is a great coach for anyone wanting to do just that. Its tests, useful exercises, and sound practical advice will help you make up the program. You need to start remembering the stuff that matters to you, from numbers, names, faces to the contents of your presentation."

—Helena Smalman-Smith, MindTools.com

"A masterful, comprehensive bible on memory and the many ways we can use associations to improve it."

—Dr. Amazing, author of *Master Your Memory with Dr. Amazing—How Not to Forget*

30 Days

to a More **POWERFUL**

Memory

Gini Graham Scott, Ph.D.

₁AMACOM

American Management Association

New York • Atlanta • Brussels • Chicago • Mexico City • San Francisco
Shanghai • Tokyo • Toronto • Washington, D.C.

Special discounts on bulk quantities of AMACOM books are available to corporations, professional associations, and other organizations. For details, contact Special Sales Department, AMACOM, a division of American Management Association, 1601 Broadway, New York, NY 10019.
Tel: 212-903-8316. Fax: 212-903-8083.
E-mail: specialsls@amanet.org
Website: www. amacombooks.org/go/specialsales
To view all AMACOM titles go to: www.amacombooks.org

Library of Congress Cataloging-in-Publication Data

Scott, Gini Graham.
      30 days to a more powerful memory / Gini Graham Scott.
         p.   cm.
      Includes bibliographical references and index.
      ISBN-13: 978-0-8144-7445-7
      ISBN-10: 0-8144-7445-4
      1. Mnemonics.   2. Memory.   I. Title.   II. Title: Thirty days to a more powerful memory.

BF385.S36   2007
153.1'4—dc22
                                                                      2006032832

Printing number

10   9   8   7   6   5   4   3   2   1

Dedicated to the many people who gave me suggestions on how to remember, including Felix Herndon, who invited me to sit in on his Cognitive Processes class at Cal State, East Bay—a source of much inspiration for many of the memory principles described in the book.

Contents

Introduction

Everyone wants a better memory—and in today's information-filled, multitasking age, having a good memory is more important than ever. Whether you need to keep track of your e-mail messages, impress the boss, give a speech, organize a busy social schedule, remember whom you met where and when, or anything else, a good memory is a necessary tool for staying on top of things. It's especially critical if you're part of the Baby Boomer generation or older, because memory loss can accompany aging. But if you keep your mind and memory limber, you can rev up your memory power—in fact, it'll even get better with age!

30 Days to a More Powerful Memory is designed to help anyone improve his or her memory. Besides drawing on the latest findings from brain and consciousness researchers, psychologists, and others about what works and why, I've included a variety of hands-on techniques and exercises, such as memory-building games and mental-imaging techniques.

While some chapters deal with basic ways of preparing your mind and body to remember more, such as improving your overall health and well-being, the main focus is on the techniques you can use day to day to improve your memory. Plus I've included chapters on creating systems so you have memory triggers or you can reduce what you have to remember, so you can concentrate on remembering what's most important to you. For example, you might feel overwhelmed if you have 20 tasks to keep in mind for a meeting; but if you organize these by priority or groups of different types of tasks and write down these categories, you might have a more manageable organization of activities to remember.

It's also important to personalize developing your memory, so you work on increasing your abilities in areas that are especially meaningful for you. By the same token, it helps to assess where you are now to figure out what you are good at remembering and where there are gaps, so you can work on those areas. Keeping a memory journal as you go through the learning process will help you track your progress, and will help you notice what you forgot, so you can work on improving your weak spots as well.

Since this is a book on improving your memory in 30 days, you should focus on committing a 30-day period to working with these techniques. You don't necessarily have to read the chapters in a particular order. In fact, you may want to spend more time on certain chapters and skip others. That's fine, but the way you use your memory is a kind of habit, and it generally takes about three weeks to form a new habit or get rid of an old one, plus an extra week thrown in for good measure. So this 30-day period will be a time when you hone new memory skills and make them a regular part of your life. With some practice, you will find that these techniques become an everyday part of your life, so you don't even have to think about them. You will just use them automatically to help you remember more.

I've also included a few introductory chapters that describe how the brain works and the different types of memory that create a memory system. This is a little like having a memory controller in charge as you take new information into your working or short-term memory, decide what bits of memory you want to keep and include in your long-term memory, and later seek to find and retrieve the memories you want. But again the focus is on using what you have learned to better apply the techniques that incorporate those principles. You'll also see helpful tips from people I have interviewed on how they remember information in different situations, and I have included examples of how I apply these techniques myself. Some of these techniques are memory games that I have developed to make increasing your memory fun. While the focus is on using these memory skills for work and professional development, you can use these skills in your personal life, too.

Back in high school and college, it was always a struggle for me to remember details. When I took a class in acting in my junior year, I found it especially difficult to remember my lines. Later on, I still had difficulty remembering things. For example, if someone asked me to repeat something I had just said—such as when I was being interviewed for a TV show or teaching a class—I could never remember it exactly, though I could answer the question anew. Yet, looking back, I can remember quite vividly my struggles to remember, even imagining where I was, the appearance of the room, and the like. That's the way memory works. When you have images, when something is more important for you, when you use multiple senses to encode the experience in the first place—when you don't just try to recall words on a page or a series of spoken words—you will remember more.

Over the years, I learned specific ways to enable me to remember things better. Now, since I have been working on this book, I have found even more techniques to improve my memory. I think you'll find the same thing as you read through the chapters.

So get ready, get set—mark your calendar and get started on improving your memory over the next 30 days. Of course, you're also free to condense the program into fewer days or extend the process if necessary. Thirty days is optimal—but adapt the program so it's best for you.

1

How Your Memory Works

To know how to improve your memory, it helps to have a general understanding of how your memory works. I have created specific exercises based on this knowledge, exercises that will help you improve in each of the areas of your memory.

The roots for the way we think about memory today actually have a long history, dating at least back to the time of the Greeks, and perhaps earlier. Accordingly, I have included a little history about the way psychologists have thought about memory that has developed into the model of memory that psychologists commonly hold today and that I use in this book.

A Quick Historical Overview

The Beginnings of Studying Memory

Even before philosophers and other theorists began to study human thought processes, including memory, memory played an extremely important part in the development of human society. It was critical for teaching new skills, customs, and traditions. Before the development of printing, people had to remember many things that now are recorded on the printed page or can be shared through audio and video recordings. For example, consider all of the rituals, songs, and stories that people had to learn and then pass on to others. This

1

ning the contents of dozens of books. Anthropolo-
ed the extensive scope of such learning by speak-
ture bearers of once nonliterate cultures and
what kind of learning might have been passed on

Then, to skip ahead to about 2,300 years ago, the Greek philoso-
pher Aristotle was one of the first to systematically study learning
and memory. Besides proposing laws for how memory works, he also
described the importance of using mental imagery, along with experience and observation—all of which are key aids for remembering
anything.

However, the formal study of memory by psychologists didn't
begin until the late 19th century, when Wilhelm Wundt set up a
laboratory in Leipzig, Germany, and launched the discipline of psychology, based on studying mental processes through introspection
or experimental studies.[1] There, along with studying other mental
processes, he began the first studies of human memory.

Many of these memory studies used assorted clinical trials,
which may seem a far cry from the practical tips on memory that are
described in this book. But the work of these researchers helped to
discover the principles of how we remember that provide the theoretical foundation for what works in effective memory training
today. For example, back in 1894, one of the first memory researchers—and the first woman president of the American Psychological
Association, Mary Whiton Calkins—discovered the recency effect,
the principle that we more accurately recall the last items we learn.[2]
These early researchers generally used nonsense syllables to determine what words a person would best remember after a series of
tests of seeing words and trying to recall them, but the recency principle still applies when you try to remember something in day-to-day
life. Want to better remember something? Then, learn it or review it
last when you are learning a series of things at the same time.

The well-known psychologist William James was also interested
in memory, discussing it in his 1890 textbook *Principles of Psychology*,
along with many of the cognitive functions that contribute to memory, such as perception and attention. He even noted the "tip-of-the-

tongue" experience that we have all had: trying to recall a name that seems so close—but not quite able to grasp it.[3]

During the first half of the 20th century the behaviorists, with their focus on outward, observable behaviors and the stimuli contributing to different behaviors, dominated psychological research in the United States. They weren't interested in mental processes or in introspection about them, though their methods of measurement were later adopted by memory researchers.[4]

But in Europe, in the early 1900s, Gestalt psychology got its start. It brought a new perspective of looking at meaning and at the way humans organize what they see into patterns and wholes. They pointed up the importance of the overall context for learning and problem solving, too.[5] It's an approach that is very relevant for understanding ways to improve memory; their work helped us understand that by creating patterns and providing a meaningful context to stimulate better encoding of a memory in the first place, that memory could more easily be retrieved later. For example, Frederick C. Bartlett, a British psychologist, who published *Remembering: An Experimental and Social Study* in 1932, who used "meaningful material" such as long stories (rather than random words or nonsense syllables), found that people made certain *types* of errors in trying to recall these stories for the researchers. Significantly, these were errors that often made the material more consistent with the subject's personal experience, showing the way meaning shapes memory.[6] Like the recency findings discussed above, these findings—that you will remember something better if you can relate it to your own experience—are the basis for some of the techniques described later in the book.

Modern Research on Memory

According to psychologists, building on the work of these early precursors, cognitive psychology—the study of mental processes, including memory—really begins in 1956. So the foundations of modern memory research only go back 50 years. As Margaret W. Matlin writes in *Cognition,* an introduction to cognitive psychology, initially published in 1983 and now in its sixth edition, "research in human memory began to blossom at the end of the 1950s. . . . Psychologists examined the organization of memory, and they proposed memory models."[7] They found that the information held in memory was frequently changed by what people previously knew or experienced—a principle that can also be applied in improving your memory. For example, if you can tie a current memory into something you already know or an experience you have previously had, you can remember more.

For a time, psychologists studying memory used an information-processing model developed by Richard Atkinson and Richard Shiffrin in 1968 that came to be known as the Atkinson-Shiffrin model. While some early memory improvement programs were based on this model, it has since been replaced by a new model that is discussed in the next section.

In the Atkinson-Shiffrin model, memory is viewed as a series of distinct steps, in which information is transferred from one memory storage area to another.[8] As this model suggests, the external input comes into the sensory memory from all of the senses—mostly visual and auditory, but also from the touch, taste, and smell—where it is stored for up to two seconds and then quickly disappears unless it is transferred to the next level. This next level is the short-term memory (now usually referred to as "working memory"), which stores information we are currently using actively for up to about 30 seconds. Finally, if you rehearse this material, such as by saying the information over and over in your mind, it goes on into the long-term memory storage area, where it becomes fairly permanent.[9]

Thus, if you want to improve your own memory, it is critical to rehearse any information you want to transfer into your long-term memory and thereby retain. Such rehearsal can take the form of self-talk, where you say the ideas to remember over and over again in your mind to implant them in your long-term memory. Graphically, this process of moving memory from sensory to short-term to long-term memory looks something like this:

| Sensory Memory | ⇨ | Short-Term Memory | ⇨ | Long-Term Memory |

Current Thinking on Memory

While the Atkinson-Shiffrin model was extremely popular at the time, today psychologists think of sensory memory as a part of perception, held only so briefly in consciousness, and they think of short-term and long-term memory as more part of a continuum, with no clear distinction between them.[10] Still, psychologists usually distinguish between these two types of memory, and I will too, in discussing ways you can improve both types of memory. In fact, with the development of neuroscience and the recognition that we are engaging in multiple forms of mental processing at the same time—a process called "parallel distributed processing"—psychologists have recognized that memory is much more complex than earlier scientists might have thought. Currently, the commonly accepted model views memory in a more dynamic way, in which a central processing system coordinates different types of memory input, which may be visual or auditory or both. After taking into consideration personal knowledge and experience, this central processor passes selected bits of memory from the working memory into the long-term memory. It's a model that I'll be using as a backdrop to different types of memory techniques that are designed to make improvements in each area of processing. In the next section, I'll explain in a little more detail how this works.

Understanding the Process

From Perception to Working Memory to Long-Term Memory

Memory starts with an initial perception as you are paying attention to something, whether your attention is barely registering the perception or you are really focused on it. So, as described in Chapter 5, one of the keys to improving your memory is paying more attention in the first place.

The next stop is your working memory, which is your brief, initial memory of whatever you are currently processing. A part of this working memory acts as a central processor or coordinator to organize your current mental activities.[11] You might think of the process as having a screen on your computer that has the information you are currently reading or writing. As psychologist Margaret Matlin explains it, your "working memory lets you keep information active and accessible, so that you can use it in a wide variety of cognitive tasks."[12] Your working memory decides what type of information is useful to you now, drawing this out from the very large amount of information you have—in your long-term memory or from the input you have recently received. Think of yourself sitting in front of a desk with expansive drawers representing what's in your long-term memory and a cluttered top of your desk representing what's in your working memory. Then, you as the central executive (the working memory) decide what information you want to deal with now and what to do with it.

The Power of Your Working Memory

How much information can you actually hold in your working memory—what can you deal with on your desktop at one time? Well, when researchers began studying the working memory, they came up with some of the findings that are still accepted and incorporated into models of memory today.

One of these findings is the well-known Magic Number Seven principle, which was first written about by George Miller in 1956 in an article titled "The Magical Number Seven, Plus or Minus Two: Some Limits on Our Capacity for Processing Information." He suggested that we can only hold about seven items, give or take two—or five to nine items—in our short-term memory (which was the term originally used for the working memory). However, if you group items together into what Miller calls "chunks"—units of short-term memory composed of several strongly related components—you can remember more.[13] And in Chapter 12 you'll learn more about how to do your own chunking to improve your memory capacity.

You can see examples of how this Number Seven principle and chunking work if you consider your phone number and social security number. One reason the phone number was originally seven numbers and divided into two groups of numbers is because of this principle—then when the area code was added, the phone number was split up or chunked into three sections. Similarly, your social security number is divided into three chunks. And when you look at your bank account, you'll see that number is chunked up into several sections. As for memory experts who can reel off long strings of numbers, they do their own mental chunking so they can remember. They don't have a single, very long string of numbers in their mind.

However you chunk it, though, whatever material comes into your working or short-term memory is frequently forgotten if you hold it in your memory for less than a minute[14]—a finding repeatedly confirmed by hundreds of studies by cognitive psychologists. That's why you normally have to do something to make that memory memorable if you want to retain it.

Yet, while you want to improve your memory for things you want to remember, you don't want to try to improve it for everything. Otherwise your mind would be so hopelessly cluttered, you would have trouble retrieving what you want. For example, think of the many activities and thoughts you experience each day, many of them part of a regular routine. Well, normally, you don't want to remember the minutia of all that, lest you drown in an overwhelming flood of perceptual data. It would be like having an ocean of memories, where the small memory fish you want to catch easily slip away and get lost in the vast watery expanses. But if something unusual happens—say a robber suddenly appears in the bank where you are about to a make a deposit—then you do want to remember the event accurately. So that's when it's important to focus and pay attention in order to capture that particular memory, much like reeling in a targeted fish.

Memory researchers have also found that your short-term or working memory is affected by when you get information about something, which is called the "serial position effect." In general, whatever type of information you are trying to memorize, you will better remember what you first learn (called the "primacy effect") or what you learn most recently (called the "recency effect").[15] When psychologists have tested these effects by giving numerous subjects lists of words that vary in word length and the number of words, the results show a similar pattern. Subjects can generally remember two to seven items and are most likely to remember the most recent items first. In turn, you can use that principle when you want to remember a list of anything, from a grocery list to a list of tasks to do.

Some Barriers to Remembering

Researchers have found that there are some cognitive barriers to a better memory that will slow you down. One is having longer names or words, especially when they have odd spellings and many syllables. Even trying to take a mental picture of the name or word may not work, because saying it verbally to yourself is an important part of putting a new name or word into your memory.

For example, I found the long words and names a real stumbling block when I tried to learn Russian two times—once when I was still in college, and later when I was taking occasional classes at a community college in San Francisco. I could even manage seeing the words in Cyrillic, converting them into their English sound equivalent. But once the words grew to more than seven or eight letters, I had to slow down to sound out each syllable and it was a real struggle to remember. Had I known the principle of chunking back then, I'm sure I would have caught on much sooner.

Another barrier to memory is interference; if some other name, word, or idea that you already have in your working memory is similar to what you are learning, it can interfere with your remembering something new correctly. And the more similar the two items, the greater the interference[16] and the more likely you are to mix them up. Again, researchers have come to these conclusions by looking at words (or even nonsense words) and pictures, and asking subjects to remember these items after learning a series of similar items. But you can take steps to keep what you have learned before from interfering with what you learn in the future. As you'll discover in Chapter 5 on paying attention, you can stop the interference by intensely focusing on what you want to remember and turning your attention away from what is similar and interfering with your memory now.

The Four Components of Your Working Memory

I have been describing the working memory as a single thing—like a temporary storage box. In fact, cognitive psychologists today think of the memory as having several components, and you can work on making improvements for each of these components to improve the initial processing of items in your memory. You might think of this process as fine-tuning the different components in a home entertainment system. For optimal quality and enjoyment, you need to fully coordinate your big-screen television, VCR, DVD, cable or satellite hookup, and sound system.

According to this current working memory model, which was developed by Alan Baddeley in 2000, there are four major components that together enable you to hold several bits or chunks of information in your mind at the same time, so your mind can work on this information and then use it.[17] Commonly, these bits of information will be interrelated, such as when you are reading a sentence and need to remember the beginning before you get to the end—though as a sentence gets longer and more complicated, you may find that you are losing the sense of it, especially if you get distracted while you are reading. But sometimes you might juggle some disparate bits of information, such as when you are driving and trying to remember where to turn off at the same time that you are having a conversation with a friend. Another example of this juggling is when you use your working memory to do mental arithmetic, like when you are balancing a checkbook; thinking about a problem and trying to figure out how to solve it; or following a discussion at a meeting and comparing what one person has just argued with what someone else said before.

The four key working memory components are coordinated by a kind of manager called the "central executive," which is in charge of the other three components: the "visuospatial sketchpad," the "episodic buffer," and the "phonological loop." Since they work independently of each other, you can handle a series of different memory tasks at the same time, such as remembering a visual image at the same time that you remember something you are listening to. You might think of these separate components as all part of a workbench that processes any information coming into it, such as the perceptions from the senses and any long-term memories pulled out of storage. Then, your working memory variously handles, combines, or transforms this material and passes some of these materials it has worked on into your long-term memory.[18] So one way to improve your memory is to improve the ability of each of these elements of your working memory to process information so that you can more effectively and efficiently send the information you want into your long-term memory.

A chart of these four components of your working memory, which is based on Alan Baddeley's working memory model, looks something like this[19]:

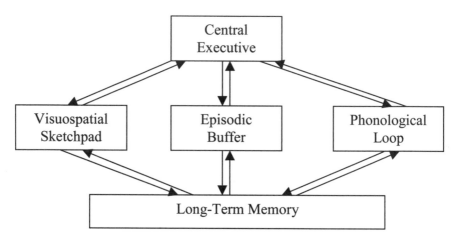

So what exactly do these four components do? Here's the latest scoop on what modern psychologists are thinking:

1. *Your Visuospatial Sketchpad.* Consider this a drawing pad in which you place visual images as you see something or where you sketch the images you create in your mind when someone tells you something.[20] For example, as you watch a TV show or movie, the series of images you see get placed on this sketchpad, and some of the most memorable will move on to your long-term memory. You won't remember every detail, since there are thousands of such images zipping by in a minute. But your memory for these images will string them together—and as you improve your memory for visual details, you will be able to notice and remember more.

This is also the section of your memory that works on turning what you are hearing or thinking about into visual images. For example, as you read or hear a story, this is where you create images for what you are listening to, so it becomes like a movie in your mind. Or suppose you are trying to work out a math problem in your mind. This is where you would see the numbers appear, such as if you are trying to multiply 24×33 and don't already have a multiplication table for that problem in your mind. You would see the individual rows as you multiply and then add them together.

However, while you might be able to see and keep in memory one image very well, you will have less ability as the number of images increase, and you may find that one image interferes with another. For example, if you are driving while trying to think about and visualize the solution to some kind of problem, your thoughts could well interfere with your driving. I found this out for myself when I was trying to multiply some numbers in my mind and took the wrong turn-off because I was distracted by seeing the problem in my mind. But if you are only listening to music on the radio or to someone speaking without forming images, that will not interfere—or at least to the same degree.

You might think of this process of trying to work with more and more images at the same time as looking at the windows on a computer screen. As you add more windows to work with at the same time, the individual windows get smaller and smaller, as do the images; you are less able to see what is in each image distinctly, and your attention to one window may be distracted by what is flashing by in another.

Intriguingly, brain researchers (also called neuroscientists) have found that these images you see in your visuospatial sketchpad correspond to real places in your brain. As neuroscientists have found, when you work with a visual image, it activates the right hemisphere of your cortex, the top section of your brain, and in particular they activate the occipital lobe, at the rear of your cortex. Then, as you engage in some mental task involving this image, your frontal lobe will get in on the action, too.

Researchers have been able to tell what part of the brain is associated with different types of thinking by using PET (positron emission tomography) scans, where they measure the blood flow to the brain by injecting a person with a radioactive chemical just before they perform some kind of mental task. They find that certain sections of the brain have more blood flow, indicating more activity there for different types of mental tasks.

2. *Your Phonological Loop.* Just as your visuospatial sketchpad stores images briefly while you are working with them, your phonological loop stores a small number of sounds for a brief period.[21] Generally, researchers have found that you can hold about as many words as you can mentally pronounce to yourself in 1.5 seconds, so you can remember more short words than long ones.[22]

A good example of how this works is when you are trying to remember what you or someone else has just said. Without memory training to put those words in long-term memory, you will normally only be able to clearly remember back what has been said in the last 1.5 seconds, though you will remember the gist of what you or the other person has said. Also, because of this 1.5-second limit, you will be better able to remember more shorter names than longer ones, such as when you are introduced to a number of people at a business mixer or cocktail party. It's simply much easier to remember names like Brown and Cooper than longer and more unusual ones.

You'll also find that just as working with different types of visual imagery can cause interference, so can working with different types of audio sounds. For example, if you are trying to remember a phone number and someone says something to you, that can interfere with your ability to remember that number. But if you are looking at something while you are trying to remember the number, that won't interfere as long as you continue to pay attention to remembering that number, since your visual observation is processed in your visuospatial sketchpad.

Then, too, just as similar visual imagery can cause memory errors, so can hearing similar sounding words or numbers, such as when you find yourself meeting a Margaret, Maggie, and Mary at a party. The names can blend together in your mind and you have trouble remembering who is who. Or say you are trying to remember a phone number you have gotten from a message so you can write it down. Well, if you are given two phone numbers to remember—such as this is my land line and this is my cell phone—the two numbers can interfere with each other, so you might mix up numbers or just not remember at all. Or if you are trying to recall and write down a number that's close to another phone number you already know, that could interfere with your ability to remember the new one.

But the reason that visual images won't interfere with trying to remember words or other audio sounds, as long as you are attending to both, is that the audio processing occurs in a different section of your brain—in the left hemisphere of your brain, which is the side of your brain that handles language. Plus the auditory information is stored in the parietal lobe of your brain, though when you practice working with this information, your frontal lobe section that processes speech will become active too.[23]

3. *Your Episodic Buffer.* This section of your working memory is essentially a temporary storehouse where you can collect and combine information that you have gotten from your visuospatial sketchpad and phonological loop, along with your long-term memory.[24] Think of this like a notebook or page in a word processing program where you are working with sentences, graphic images, and then thinking about what else you would like to add from what you already know. As Margaret Matlin describes it, the episodic buffer "actively manipulates information so that you can interpret an earlier experience, solve new problems, and plan future activities."[25]

For example, say a co-worker says something to you at work that offends you. This is where you might consider the words the person just said, the context in which he said it, and take into consideration what you remember from how this co-worker has acted toward you before (which comes from your long-term memory). Then, this episodic buffer helps you quickly decide what to do in light of how you have interpreted this offending remark.

4. *Your Central Executive.* Finally, your central executive pulls together and integrates the information from these three other systems—the visuospatial sketchpad, the phonological loop, and the episodic buffer. In addition, this executive function helps to determine where you are going to place your attention and suppresses irrelevant or unimportant information, so you can stay focused on

what's important and not be distracted by what isn't. It also helps you plan strategies and coordinate behavior, so you decide what to do next and what not to do. Then you don't get pulled away from what you most want to do.[26]

Think of this as the top executive or senior manager in charge of all of these other systems, which doesn't store information itself. Rather, like the executive of a company, it sets the priorities for what these other sections of your memory should be doing. Or as Matlin puts it: "like an executive supervisor in an organization . . . the [central] executive decides which issues deserve attention and which should be ignored. The executive also selects strategies, figuring out how to tackle a problem."[27]

For example, when you decide what task you are going to work on at work and seek to remember what your boss has instructed you to do, along with what else you know about how to best perform the task, that's your central executive pulling together what is most relevant from the other sections of your working and long-term memory, so you can better perform the task.

* * *

So there you have it—the basic structure of how your memory works, according to the latest research from cognitive psychologists. In subsequent chapters, I'll be drawing on this model as I describe different techniques for optimizing your memory. Accordingly, you'll find techniques for strengthening your ability to work with images (your visuospatial sketchpad), with verbal and audio input (your phonological loop), with your ability to temporarily coordinate the input from the other components of your memory (your episodic buffer), and with your ability to use all of this information in a mindful, coordinated, and strategic way (your central executive).

2

How Your Long-Term Memory Works

In the last chapter, I described how your working short-term memory takes in new information and then passes some of it on to your long-term memory. In this chapter, I'll describe how your long-term memory works, so you will better understand the techniques used for putting information into your long-term memory—and later, retrieving information from there. Again I have drawn on the latest findings from cognitive psychologists in writing this chapter.

You might think of your long-term memory as akin to a hard drive on a computer, whereas your working memory is like your RAM (random access memory), which you use in processing current tasks and which has only a limited space. Your long-term memory is very large, and contains everything you've ever put into it, from experiences to images and information. You may have to do some digging around to find specific information. Sometimes, as when you're struggling to recall something you haven't thought about for a very long time, you may think certain information has been deleted, but it may well be there if you know how to retrieve it.

The Three Types of Long-Term Memory

Commonly, psychologists divide long-term memory into three types of memory, although this may be more of a convenience for thinking about how we remember than actual distinctions. However, different techniques will help you improve in each of these areas, so these distinctions have practical uses.

These three types of memory include episodic, semantic, and procedural memory, which have the following characteristics discussed below.[1]

Episodic Memory

This is your memory for experiences or events that happened to you at any time in the past—from many years ago to just a few minutes ago. When you call up these memories, you travel backwards in time so you can experience what happened in the past—or at least what you remember happened, since this recollection is subjective.[2] Thus, someone else might have a different memory of what happened and a video recording might show a still different reality. So while your memory may well be accurate, it is also subject to distortion for various reasons, such as your faulty encoding of this memory in the first place or a later modification of the memory to conform to your self-perception of how you are now. Then, too, your memory might be modified by later suggestions about what you experienced; this sometimes happens in conversations and interviews, as when a cop interviews a witness or suspect with leading questions that shape what the person remembers. (You'll see some techniques for how to more accurately pull up these memories in Chapters 24 and 26.)

Semantic Memory

This is your memory for what you know about the world. It is like an organized base of knowledge; it includes any factual or other information you have learned, including all the words you know in any language.[3] You might think of this semantic memory as your internal encyclopedia or reference desk, which you are continually consulting as you speak, read the newspaper, listen to the radio or TV, or consider the validity of new information from any source. And just as your episodic memory can be faulty at times, so can your semantic memory.

Procedural Memory

This is your memory for your knowledge about how to do something.[4] Commonly, once this knowledge gets transferred into your long-term memory it becomes automatic. You don't have to think about driving a car, for example, or opening up a word-processing program and starting to type. But like any skill, if you don't use it, you can forget exactly what you are doing, much like any unused mechanical device might become rusty or a computer program might become corrupted and stop working properly.

Encoding Your Memories

Regardless of which type of memory you are placing in long-term memory, the transfer process from working to long-term memory depends on encoding—the action of placing a particular bit of information there. The process is a little like placing a file folder, in which you have just placed some documents, into a file cabinet.

The more carefully you place it there and the more clearly you identify what's in that file, the better you will be able to retrieve it later. In fact, psychologists distinguish between two types of encoding: psychologists call this the "levels-of-processing" or "depth-of-processing." You can either encode something through a more shallow type of encoding or a deeper level of processing.[5] The difference affects your ability to retrieve information later.

When you use a more shallow type of processing, you are essentially using your *senses* to place the information in long-term memory. For example, you are focusing on the way a word or image looks or sounds. In the tests psychologists use for testing memory, this appearance or sound might be distinguished by whether a word is typed in capital or small letters, rhymes with another word, or comes before or after another word in a sequence. In the case of an image, your focus would be on its appearance, such as its shape, color, or identity. Or in everyday life, you might do shallow processing when you remember someone by his or her facial features or what he or she is wearing.

By contrast, when you use a deep processing approach, you are looking at the *meaning* of something. For instance, if it's a word, you might think of whether it fits in a sentence or what types of images and associations it brings to mind. If it's an image, you would think about its associations, too. And in everyday life, you would seek to remember more details about someone beyond his or her superficial appearance, such as his or her occupation, where and how you met, and your thoughts about how you might be able to have a mutually profitable relationship in the future.

As psychologists have found, when you use deep processing to remember something, you will better recall it later. Why? Because of two key factors: (1) making the information more distinctive and (2) elaborating on it.[6] For example, you might make the name of someone you have just met more distinctive by identifying something unusual about that name or thinking about how that person is unique, such as if that person has an unusual occupation. Or you might elaborate on some new information by thinking about how it connects to something else you already know or about its meaning and significance, such as when you read a news article and think about the impact that an event discussed in the article will have.

In addition, psychologists have discovered three other factors that contribute to deeper encoding and therefore better retrieval: (1) the self-referent effect, (2) the power of context and specificity, and (3) the influence of the emotions and mood. Moreover, psychologists have found that these deeper encoding processes make more of an impact within the brain itself than shallower processing. For example, they have found that when subjects in experiments engage in deep processing, they activate the left prefrontal cortex, which is associated with verbal and language processing.[7] This deep processing approach has also been found to be especially effective in trying to remember faces, by paying more attention to the distinctions between features and consciously trying to recall more facial features.[8]

You'll see more about techniques that are based on each of these factors in subsequent chapters. But for now, here's how these different factors contribute to better remembering something.

Using the Self-Referent Effect for a Better Memory

The way the self-referent effect works is that if you can relate the information to yourself, you will better remember it. Psychologists have found this association again and again, when they have asked subjects to decide if a particular word could apply to themselves, rather than just trying to remember the word based on how it looks or sounds, or on its meaning.[9] One reason is that as you think about how something relates to you, you make it more distinctive and you elaborate on what that word means to you. The same process works when you think about anything, such as how someone you have just met might be able to help you or how you might be able to use a new product you are reading about in your own life. As you think about it, you make that information more distinctive and you elaborate on it by considering what it means to you. You might also be more likely to continue to think about it, a process that psychologists call "rehearsal," as you repeatedly call up a new idea, name, or any other sort of new information.

Intriguingly, psychologists have found that this self-reference approach lights up a particular area of the brain—the right prefrontal cortex, which researchers suggest may be an area of the brain associated with the concept of self.[10] So as you use these various techniques—for deep processing—such as finding ways to increase the way a particular bit of information relates to you—it has a direct effect on your brain processing, too. No wonder these techniques work so well. You are not only creating more meanings and associations for words and relating them to yourself, but your actions are activating your brain centers involved with language and your sense of self.

Using the Power of Context and Specificity

Another way to increase your encoding ability is to incorporate the specific context, and then use that context when you seek to retrieve that memory.[11] A good example of how the power of context works is when you meet someone at an event and later you run into that person dressed differently on the street. You may not even recognize the person or you may only have a vague sense of familiarity—you think you may have seen that person before but you don't have the slightest idea where. But if the other person has a better memory for your meeting and mentions where you met, the memory of who that person is may come flooding back. Why? Because you now have the context for your meeting, which cues you in to who this person is and what transpired in your meeting.

A similar kind of experience may occur when you go to get something from another room but once you get there, you don't have any idea why you are there. No, you are not suffering the early stages of Alzheimer's disease. You have simply moved out of the context in which you encoded the item and remembered why you need it. In a different context, you don't remember what you were looking for. But once you return to the original room, you will remember.

Psychologists have developed some terms that highlight the importance of context for remembering. One is the "encoding specificity principle," which means that you will better recall something if you are in a context that's similar to where you encoded the information—that is, when you entered it into your long-term memory.[12] By contrast, you are more likely to forget when you experience a different context. Two other terms that psychologists use to refer to this phenomenon are that your memory is "context-dependent" or that "transfer-appropriate processing" helps you better remember.[13] In other words, if you are having trouble remembering something, it can help to go back into the setting where you first encoded it into memory. Or if you can't actually go there, you can mentally project yourself into that setting—one of the techniques I'll discuss further in Chapters 24 and 26.

Repeatedly, psychologists have found examples of this encoding specificity principle in their research, in which memory is dependent on the context where the original memory is encoded. For example, they found that people hearing a male or female speak some words were more likely to remember the word when they heard the words spoken again by someone of the same sex.[14] They have also found that subjects will recall an earlier experience in extensive detail when triggered by a present-day stimulus that evokes that experience. For example, an image of an exotic bird you haven't seen in years brings back memories of going on a birding trip to the tropics.

While the physical context can serve as a reminder, so can the mental context, because it's not just how the environment looks but how it feels.[15] For example, you may experience an extremely hot day in one place that brings up memories of how you felt when it was extremely hot someplace else; a bitter cold day now can bring up memories of a bitter cold winter long ago.

The Influence of Emotion and Mood

Finally, cognitive psychologists have found that your emotional feelings and mood can affect what you remember. Not only is there the same kind of matching effect that there is for context, so you will remember more if you are in a similar emotional state when you try to retrieve a memory, but you will remember more if you feel the memory is a pleasant one.[16] Here are three major findings about memory, emotions, and mood.

- *You will recall pleasant information more accurately and more quickly,* which is sometimes called the "Pollyanna Principle." Whether you are trying to remember what you have perceived, what someone has said, a decision you have made, or other types of information, if it's more pleasant to remember, you will remember better. While psychologists have tested this principle in the laboratory, such as by asking subjects to remember words that are pleasant, neutral, or unpleasant, or asking them to remember colors, fruits, vegetables, or other items that are more or less pleasant,[17] the principle makes sense in everyday life. For example, wouldn't you rather recall something you enjoy that gives you good feelings than something you don't like and makes you feel bad? In fact, there is a whole body of research that indicates that people will repress or suppress memories of experiences that are unpleasant, such as memories of early childhood abuse.[18]

- *You will more accurately recall neutral information associated with pleasant information or a pleasant context,* or as psychologists phrase it, you will have "more accurate recall for neutral stimuli associated with pleasant stimuli."[19] Psychologists have come to this conclusion by making comparisons in the lab, such as whether subjects better remember commercials or the brands featured in them when they see them before or after violent and nonviolent films. Again and again, psychologists have found significantly better recall when nonviolent, and presumably more pleasant, films are shown.[20] The finding makes perfect sense and you can see examples of how this works in everyday life. For example, when you are experiencing or seeing something pleasant, you will feel more comfortable and relaxed, which will contribute to your remembering something you read, hear, or perceive in this relaxed state. By contrast, if you are experiencing something unpleasant, you will feel more stress and tension; the experience may even interfere with your ability to concentrate, such as by distracting your attention, so you encode and remember less.

- *You will retain your pleasant memories longer, while unpleasant memories will fade faster.* It's a principle some researchers discovered when they asked subjects to record personal events for about three months and rate how pleasant they were, and three months later, asked them to rate the events again. While there was little change for the neutral and pleasant events, most of the subjects rated the less pleasant events as more pleasant when they recalled them again. The one unexpected finding was that if subjects tended to feel depressed, they were more likely to better recall the unpleasant memories.[21] But this finding makes sense when you think about it. You are more likely to focus on and remember the experiences you have found pleasant in your life, since they will make you feel better. But if you are unhappy, you will be more likely to recall the negative, unpleasant experiences you have had, though these will contribute to keeping you feeling down.

Cognitive psychologists have additionally found that just as there is improved memory when the context matches, so there is a match between what you remember and your mood. If you are in a good mood, you will remember pleasant material better than unpleasant material, while if you are in a bad mood, you will better remember unpleasant material. Likewise, if you are a generally upbeat person, your memory for positive information will be greater than the memory of someone who tends to be down and depressed. In turn, these positive memories will help keep someone who is positive upbeat, while a depressed person could become even more down in the dumps as they remember more negative memories.[22] In other words, as the old popular song puts it: "accentuate the positive" in what you think about and remember if you want to feel better.

Retrieving Your Memories

Once a memory is encoded in long-term memory, there are several ways to retrieve it—and many of the techniques described in later chapters will help you do that.

Psychologists distinguish between two ways of looking at how well you retrieve a memory—either *explicitly* through recall or recognition, or *implicitly*, when your memory enables you to do some activity, even though you aren't consciously trying to remember how to do it.[23]

Your recall is your ability to call up a particular memory; your recognition is your ability to recognize whether or not you know or are familiar with something. As you well know from your own experience, it's always more difficult to recall something than to simply recognize it as being familiar. This is the difference between having to come up with a definition or identification for something on a test versus selecting a multiple-choice or true/false answer.

One way that psychologists test for recall ability—an approach that will be incorporated in some later exercises for memory improvement—is asking subjects to read a list of words, then take a break, and later try to write down as many words as they can. Or they might do this exercise with numbers, nonsense syllables, cities, animal names, or anything else they choose.

They test for recognition in a very similar way. Subjects are given a list of words or other items and, after a break, are shown another list and asked to identify the items on the original list.[24] In both recall and recognition, errors can easily creep in, such as not remembering an item on a list or thinking that something is on the list that isn't.

As for implicit memory, a typical example of testing for this ability is to give subjects in an experiment a list of items with some information left out—such as having missing letters in words or having some missing lines in a drawing.[25] Then, the subjects have to fill in what's missing. If they have seen the words, drawings, or other items in the test before, they will be able to complete the items more quickly and accurately, because they have a memory of seeing those items before.

Whatever the type of task, if you have previous experience with the material or skill involved, you will be able to do it better. For example, even if you haven't ridden a bike, picked up a tennis racquet, or spoken a language you learned in college for many years, you will generally find if you are in a situation where you have to use that skill again, you will be able to use it even if you are a little rusty. When you work on learning and remembering that ability again, you will learn it faster than you did the first time.

Moreover, if your experience is more recent, you will be more likely to recall, recognize, or use an implicit memory to complete a task. So it makes sense to refresh your memory closer to the time when you will need it—otherwise, a good recollection of something may not be there when you need it. For example, a woman in a Native American literature class I took thought she would get a leg up on the course if she read over the material the first night after the class. But when it came time to take a short quiz on the reading, she completely blanked out on the stories. However, when the professor discussed the books later in the course, she found the material familiar.

That loss of memory is what happens if you learn something too far away in time from when you need to recall that information and don't try to refresh your memory closer to the time you need to know this material. Your memory of something you have learned gradually fades if you don't use that memory. So while you may be able to recognize that you learned something days later or may be able to pull up relevant information with a specific trigger word, phrase, or sentence, a more general recall task will leave you blank. As you'll learn in subsequent chapters, there are strategies to use in order to freshen up selective memories and decide when to learn what you need to know.

Another complication to storing and retrieving new information is that when you learn something, what you have previously learned may interfere with learning something new. Psychologists call this "proactive interference"—and there can be even more interference when the two things you are trying to learn are similar.[26] Your previous memories interfere with what you are learning now. For instance, you meet a woman named Angie at a party and you already know an Annie—you might mistakenly call Angie, Annie, and even if you are corrected, you may continue to make that same mistake. Or say you are trying to learn about the new regulations affecting your insurance policy. You may find your memory of the old policy interfering, so you confuse the two. Improving your memory will help you deal with this proactive interference problem. Incidentally, don't confuse proactive interference, which is a problem when past learning interferes with future learning, with proactive listening and observing, which is something you want to do so you more actively learn something when you listen or look closely.

How Do the Experts Do It?

Given all these difficulties in retrieving a memory correctly—from improper coding and distortion to interference from previous memories—how do the memory experts do it? What tricks and techniques do they use to make them so much better?

First of all, if it makes you feel any better, experts are generally experts in a particular area, where they have studied the subject matter intensively. In other words, most experts gain their skill through extensive training and practice. As Matlin notes of the many experts studied who have great memories for chess, sports, maps, and musical notations, "In general, researchers have found a strong positive correlation between knowledge about an area and memory performance in that area . . . [and] people who are expert in one area seldom display outstanding general memory skills."[27] For example, researchers have found that chess masters may be experts in remembering chess positions and some are even able to hold the positions on multiple boards in their head, but they are similar to nonexperts in their general cognitive and perceptual abilities. Moreover, memory experts don't have exceptionally high scores on intelligence tests. Researchers even found that one horse racing expert only had an IQ of 92 and an eighth-grade education.[28]

Rather, what makes these memory experts so good at what they do is that they have become especially knowledgeable and practiced in a particular area—so you can do it, too. In particular, researchers have found that memory experts have these key traits—and you'll find some techniques drawn from these findings in later chapters.

- Memory experts have a well-organized structure of knowledge, which they have carefully learned in a particular field.[29]

- The experts generally use more vivid imagery to help them remember.

- The experts are more likely to organize any new material they have to recall into organized and meaningful chunks of information.

- The experts use special rehearsal techniques when they practice, such as focusing on particular words or images that are likely to help them remember the rest of that material; they don't try to remember everything.

- The experts more effectively can fill in the blanks when they have missing information in material they have partially learned and remembered, such as when they are able to fill in the rest of a story they are recalling and recounting to others.

These techniques, in turn, work well for anyone, such as professional speakers and actors, who have to encode and remember a lot of information in their field—and these are techniques you can use, too. For example, professional actors use deeper rather than superficial processing techniques, such as thinking about the meanings and motivations of the character they are portraying. They also use visualization to see the person with whom they are talking as they practice their lines, and they try to put themselves in the appropriate mood and think about how the story relates to themselves.[30] In short, they don't just try to remember a lot of lines by rote, but they create a rich context for encoding and later retrieving the memory of their lines.

Remembering What You Experienced

Finally, there is one other area of long-term memory that has been much studied by researchers—an area that cognitive psychologists call "autobiographical memory."[31] It includes not only long-ago personal experiences, but also your observations when you witness a major event, such as a crime.

Commonly, this kind of memory includes a narrative or story about the event that you relate. But it additionally includes all sorts of elaborations that contribute to the significance of the story, such as the imagery you associate with the event and your emotional reactions to it. These memories also contribute to creating your personal identity, history, and sense of self, because they are all about what you experienced.

Researchers are especially interested in looking at how well these autobiographical memories match what really happened. In other words, is your recall correct? What is especially interesting about this type of memory is the way errors can creep in, so you have distorted memories or remember things that didn't even happen—even though your memory assures you that you really were there. You may make such mistakes for various reasons. One reason is you want to keep your memories consistent with your own current self-image or your current perceptions of the person involved. Another reason is that you may find something about the memory painful, so you would rather not recall it or want to edit out the painful parts from the past.

In general, though, as researchers have found, your memory is accurate in remembering what's central to the event. By contrast, you are more likely to make mistakes in correctly recalling less important details or specific small bits of tangential information. As Matlin notes, citing a study by R. Sutherland and H. Hayes, "When people do make mistakes, they generally concern peripheral details and specific information about commonplace events, rather than central information about important events."[32] In fact, researchers have found it's better not to try to remember a lot of small details; that's where you are more likely to make mistakes.

Such mistakes can also occur when you have what researchers call a "flashbulb memory," which occurs in a situation where you initially are involved in, learn of, or observe an event that is very unusual, surprising, or emotionally arousing. It's called a flashbulb memory because it may be especially vivid, such as a shocking event like 9/11, some especially good news, or the accidental death of someone close to you. Typically, you are likely to recall exactly where you were, what happened during the event, what you were doing when you heard the news, who told you, your own feelings about the event, and what happened afterwards. Yet, while the very vividness and distinctiveness of the incident may lead you to remember it in more detail and with more accuracy than everyday events, particularly when you talk about it more with others, think about it more, and consider how the event affects you, you may still make mistakes. One source of confusion may be the comments and reactions of others, which may shape your own experience and how you remember that experience. Then, too, many details may fade over time.

Another type of error that can creep in to any kind of autobiographical memory is what researchers call "consistency bias"—our tendency to make what happened in the past more consistent with our current feelings, beliefs, and general knowledge or expectations about the way things are.[33] This overall outlook we have for seeing the world is what cognitive psychologists call our "schema"—our generalized knowledge or expectation from past experiences with an event, object, or person that influences our perception and response now.[34] Thus, we may tend to downplay what seems inconsistent with who we are now—or who we think others to be. For example, if you really like your Aunt Mildred and think she is a cool person to be around, you may tend to diminish or forget your feelings that she used to treat you badly when you were young. Or if you have become a solid conservative citizen now, you may tend to downplay or forget many times when you were a spacey liberal activist in the past.

Thus, when you use memory recall techniques to tap into your personal autobiography, you have to pay careful attention so you can distinguish what you really do remember and what you might have added to or subtracted from your memory of that experience later.

This caution is especially applicable when it comes to eyewitness reports. You may think you have accurately seen something, but you really haven't. There's a classic test that teachers sometimes do with students where they have one or two people suddenly come into the class and do something dramatic—like one person chasing another with a gun or they have a mock fight—and then run out of the room. The teacher will then ask the students what they recall, and typically there are mistakes in identifications. The wrong person is seen holding the gun, the students think the man with the mustache is clean shaven, and so on. No wonder that researchers have found that in over half the cases where defendants have been mistakenly convicted it's because of faulty eyewitness testimony.[35]

One reason that eyewitness memories are often faulty is because of what researchers call the "misinformation effect," which occurs when people are given incorrect information about what they have observed and they later recall the incorrect information rather than what they actually saw.[36] This disruption is due to what cognitive psychologists call "retroactive interference," which occurs when recently learned new material interferes with recalling a previous memory correctly. For example, you see something very clearly, but then someone provides misinformation in asking you a question. Later you can't remember what you initially observed because you are recalling the new information, or you are confused about what you really saw.[37]

A good example of this retroactive interference is when a lawyer or cop is interviewing a witness who has seen a crime occur and asks what happened when he or she saw the person holding a gun. Maybe the accused person didn't have a gun at all, but the witness will now remember him holding a gun. And so a false memory is born. In fact, there have been cases where individuals have come to believe that they committed a crime under intensive questioning.

During the late 1970s and early 1980s, there was an explosion of false memories that occurred when individuals reported early memories of childhood abuse that they had forgotten or repressed. While some of these reports were valid, in many cases they were remembering imagined memories, sometimes suggested by therapists or because of the influence of recovered memory therapy groups. A similar situation has occurred in the more recent priest child abuse cases involving young males, where some accusers have recalled long-repressed memories while others have remembered events that never happened.

The reason for these recovered false memories is that sometimes therapists probing for reasons for a person's current problem will make suggestions while asking their questions. Then clients can come to believe that they do remember something, which memory becomes elaborated through further therapy, hypnosis, and interactions with other clients who are recovering their own memories. Indeed, cognitive psychologists are able to produce false memories in the lab. For example, they will give the subject a list containing a family of related words (such as water, stream, lake, boat, swim) and later the subject comes up with a related word (e.g., river) that wasn't on the original list.[38] So the subjects are creating their own false memories through their active imagination.

So what can you do to remember past events in your life more accurately? How do you avoid the effects of suggestion, retroactive interference, and misinformation distorting a past memory or creating a new one that you think occurred in the past? You'll see some suggested ways to improve your autobiographical memory in Chapter 17 on remembering a story, as well as in Chapters 24 and 26.

How Good Is Your Memory?

When you learn any kind of new subject or skill, to see how much you have improved, it's good to see where you started from. So this chapter is designed to provide you with a baseline showing how you feel about your ability to remember now and how you perform on different types of memory tests. Then, you can repeat the tests after you finish this book and examine the changes. You should expect to do better the second time.

These tests will give you a general idea of where you are now, though they are not scientific tests. The first test depends on your honest assessment of your memory abilities, and it depends on both your own candor and how accurately you make your assessment. If you approach the test with a similar attitude both times you take it (now and after 30 days), you should be reasonably accurate in assessing your own feelings and perceptions about your memory.

In the second set of tests, there is a problem with taking exactly the same test as a before-and-after test, because anything you remember about the first test will improve how you do on the second one. I have tried to overcome this problem by giving you *similar types* of tests to take before and after you read the book, so you can compare your score. Using the techniques you have learned, you should do better after 30 days.

Keeping those cautions in mind, here are the tests. I have drawn inspiration from the memory tests in a dozen different books on memory, but I have mostly come up with my own items. For the objective tests, there is a before-and-after set for each test. Just look at the first set you are taking—and wait until you have finished the book to take the second set. Otherwise, if you look at the second set now, you may influence your results when you take the test again and therefore any improved results won't be valid.

Self-Assessment

This first test will provide you with a baseline measure of your feelings about how good your memory skills are right now.

Test #1: Assessing Your Memory Skills

The following test is designed for you to subjectively reflect on your memory abilities now. Make an extra copy of this test, so you can answer it again after you have spent a month working on improving your memory. That way, you can monitor any improvement. The first time you take the test, answer each question as honestly as you can and total up your score. This will help you notice the areas where you especially need to work on memory improvement, such as learning to pay better attention, increasing your ability to encode information, and improving your ability to retrieve names, faces, places, and dates. Rate your memory on a scale of 1 (you forget most or all of the time) to 5 (you typically remember very well), and then obtain an average for each category (total up the ratings in that category and divide by the number in that category).

TEST #1: RATING MY MEMORY

My Overall Memory _____

My Memory for Everyday People, Places, and Things[1] _____
(average of my scores for the categories below)

People's names _____

People's faces _____

Where I put things (e.g., keys, eyeglasses) _____

Performing household chores _____

Directions to places _____

Personal dates (i.e., birthdays, anniversaries)

My Memory for Numbers _____
(average of my scores for the categories below)

Phone numbers I have just looked up _____

Phone numbers I use frequently_____

Bank account numbers _____

Computer passwords _____

Combinations for locks and safes _____

My Memory for Information _____
(average of my scores for the categories below)

Words _____

What someone has told me in a conversation _____

What I have learned in a classroom lecture _____

Reading a novel _____

Reading a nonfiction book _____

Reading an article _____

Reading the newspaper _____

My Memory for Activities _____
(average of my scores for the categories below)

Appointments _____

Performing household chores _____

Shopping for items at a store _____

Speaking in public _____

A meeting at work _____

My Memory for Events _____
(average of my scores for the categories below)

Earlier today_____

Yesterday_____

Last week _____

Last month _____

6 months to a year ago _____

1–5 years ago _____

6–10 years ago _____

When I was a child _____

After you finish rating each particular item, find the average for remembering that type of information. Then, look at your ratings to assess how well you are doing in different areas. Commonly, you will find you remember best those things that are most important to you, since you naturally pay more attention in those areas. But, where are you especially weak? Those are areas ripe for improvement.

Use this test as a guide to help you determine where you especially want to increase your memory. Later, after you have worked on developing your memory over the next month (or however long you take to do this), retest yourself without looking at how you rated yourself before. Afterwards, compare your before-and-after ratings. Generally, you will find you improve, though your subjective ratings can be affected by other factors, such as how you are feeling when you take the test.

In any case, your second set of scores can help you decide what you want to work on next if you want to continue to improve your memory. In fact, if you're into charts and graphs, you can plot your ratings every month to chart your continued progress.

Objective Tests of Your Different Memory Abilities

The following objective tests are other ways of testing your memory for different types of information. Some of these tests will also show how well you can avoid interference from similar types of information. Again, determine your scores now, and test yourself a second time in 30 days to see your progress. And if you continue to work on improving your memory, try testing yourself every 30 days. To avoid the effect of remembering what you have previously learned from a test, test yourself with an alternate version of the test (such as new sets of words and faces). You can use Set 2 for your second test or work with a friend or associate to create another version of the test for each other. (For example, ask a friend to come up with a list of 10 random words for you to remember.)

Remembering Random Words

This is a classic test that memory researchers use—you are presented with a list of random words (or words in a certain category), and then you have to recall as many as you can, or you have to recognize whether they are in another list. Here are series of word tests, and you can easily have a friend or associate come up with additional word tests for you. See how well you can do under different conditions. There are two sets—one to test yourself now, the other to test yourself later. Get a sheet of paper and a pencil to write down your answers and scores.

Test #2A: Immediate Recall

Take a minute to look at the following list of words; then close the book, and see how many you can write down correctly from your memory in a minute or two. Then, when you finish, look in the book and score 1 point for each correct word, subtract 1 point for each incorrect word, and total your score.

IMMEDIATE RECALL TEST

Set 1: To Test Yourself Now	Set 2: To Test Yourself in 30 Days
Pencil	Animal
Wood	Fox
House	Court
Book	Movie
Television	Pen
Box	Circle
Lamp	Elevator
Couch	Farm
Night	Factory
Moon	Wall

Test #2B: Delayed Recall

Now see how well you can do when you engage in another activity before testing your recall. As in the first test, take a minute to look at the following list of words, then close the book. But before you try to recall, do something else for 20 minutes. Do whatever you want, such as taking a walk, reading a newspaper, having a snack, or shooting baskets in your backyard. Just don't think about the words on the word list. Then, see how many words you can write down correctly from your memory in a minute or two. As before, when you finish, look in the book and score 1 point for each correct word, subtract 1 point for each incorrect word, and total your score. Compare your results with the immediate recall test. Generally, you will recall less than when you immediately tried to recall the words. This will give you a general sense of your ability to retain information in your working memory and how quickly you forget.

DELAYED RECALL TEST

Set 1: To Test Yourself Now	Set 2: To Test Yourself in 30 Days
Bathtub	Door
Computer	Elephant
Printer	Cow
Desk	Snow
File Cabinet	Mirror
Car	Tree
Motorcycle	Rose
Road	River
Sign	Fountain
Window	Bucket

Recognizing Words with Interference

How well can you recognize words that you saw when they are mixed in with other words that you didn't see before?

Test #3A: Immediate Recognition

Take a minute to look at the left-hand column (Set 1) of the following first list of words; then cover up these words with a sheet of paper, and look at the left-hand column of the second list, directly below it. Check off which words you just saw on the first list. When you finish, look at the first list again, score 1 point for each word you recognized correctly, subtract 1 point for each incorrect word, and total your score. At the end of 30 days, repeat the test with the words in the first list in the right-hand column (Set 2) and the words in the second list, directly below it.

IMMEDIATE RECOGNITION TEST

Set 1: To Test Yourself Now	Set 2: To Test Yourself in 30 Days
First List	*First List*
Camel	Jury
Cigarette	Building
Sword	House
Mule	Cement
Book	Flower
Floor	Timer
Garden	Pot
Tent	Stove
Post	Cord
Attic	Fireplace
Second List	*Second List*
(Which words from the first list are on this?)	*(Which words from the first list are on this?)*
Cigar	Clock
Horse	House
Garden	Jury
Stick	Oven
Floor	Fire
Post	Cord
Sword	Daisy
Wallet	Cement
Book	Ocean
Film	Pot

Test #3B: Delayed Recognition

Now how well can you recognize what you saw when they are mixed in with other words that you didn't see before when you engage in another activity before seeing what you can recognize? Take a minute to look at the left-hand column of the following first list of words; then cover up these words with a sheet of paper. But before you do the recognition test with the second list, do something else for 20 minutes. Again do whatever you want, such as taking a walk, reading a newspaper, having a snack, or shooting baskets in your backyard. Just don't think about the words on the word list. Then, for the test, look at the left-hand column of the second list directly below it and check off which words you just saw on the first list. When you finish, look at the first list again, score 1 point for each word you recognized correctly, subtract 1 point for each incorrect word, and total your score. Then, compare your results with the immediate recognition test. Generally, you will recognize less accurately than when you immediately tried to recognize the words. This will give you a general sense of your ability to retain information in your working memory and how quickly you forget. At the end of 30 days, repeat the test with the first list of words in the right-hand column (Set 2) and the words in the second list, directly below it.

DELAYED RECOGNITION TEST

Set 1: To Test Yourself Now	Set 2: To Test Yourself in 30 Days
First List	*First List*
Gun	Planet
Stairway	Rice
Campsite	Candy
Log	Frog
Branch	Stream
Paper	Hole
Notebook	Bandage
Chair	Hammer
Radio	Roof
Bank	Color

Set 1: To Test Yourself Now	Set 2: To Test Yourself in 30 Days
Second List	*Second List*
(Which words from the first list are on this?)	*(Which words from the first list are on this?)*
Rifle	Stream
Stairway	Planet

Radio	Harp
Lantern	Card
Donkey	Candy
Branch	Wind
Briefcase	Hammer
Lamp	Closet
River	Purple
Paper	Hole

Remembering Lists and Directions

Following are some tests for remembering lists, such as a shopping list, and directions. How well can you recall what's on the list? Sure you can write down what you want to remember, but what if you lose the list? Or what if someone gives you directions on the telephone and you can't write them down? Not only do you have to remember the directions themselves, but it's crucial to remember them in the proper order.

Test #4A: Lists

Take a minute to review the list and remember as much as you can. Then, close the book and write down whatever you remember in sequence. Give yourself 1 point for each item you remember on the list—until you miss an item. Take this as either an immediate recall test, or as a delayed recall test, where you do something else for 20 minutes and don't think of anything on the test. In either case, use the same timing—immediate or delayed—when you retake the test using the list in Set 2, and compare how well you did after working on memory improvement for 30 days.

LIST MEMORY TEST

Set 1: To Test Yourself Now

1. Shampoo
2. Soap
3. Hamburger

Set 2: To Test Yourself in 30 Days

1. Soup
2. Cheese
3. Sugar

4. Lettuce	4. Salt
5. Candy	5. Apples
6. Chocolate	6. Pears
7. Cheese	7. Applesauce
8. Soup	8. Honey
9. Tomatoes	9. Raisins
10. Carrots	10. Cookies
11. Mushrooms	11. Sour Cream
12. Salt	12. Milk
13. Sugar	13. Steak
14. Cocoa	14. Chicken
15. Milk	15. Peanuts

Test #4B: Directions

DIRECTIONS MEMORY TEST

Set 1: To Test Yourself Now

1. Turn off freeway.
2. Left on Franklin.
3. Right on Mildred.
4. Go 1 mile.
5. Right at 7/11.
6. Left at Wal-Mart.
7. Go 2 miles.
8. Right at Harrison.
9. Left on Williams.
10. Go to 939 Williams.

Set 2: To Test Yourself in 30 Days

1. Get onto freeway.
2. Exit at Ross.
3. Right on Thompson.
4. Left on Jackson.
5. Go $1/2$ mile.
6. Left at Sears.
7. Right at flagpole.
8. Go 1 mile.
9. Left at Henry.
10. Park at the art store.

Remembering Numbers

How good are you at remembering phone numbers, bank account numbers, passwords, and other sets of numbers and letters? Here's a chance to test yourself in the following tests, where you have an increasing number of numbers to remember. To do the test, look at the initial list for 1 minute, then close the book and try to recall as much as you can, using an immediate or delayed recall test. Write down what you recall, and afterwards compare it to what's in the book. Give yourself 1 point for each number or letter in its correct place in the sequence.

Test #5A: Phone Numbers

PHONE NUMBER RECALL TEST—1

Set 1: To Test Yourself Now	Set 2: To Test Yourself in 30 Days
510-798-3423	798-325-3512
324-803-9241	867-441-7654

PHONE NUMBER RECALL TEST—2

Set 1: To Test Yourself Now	Set 2: To Test Yourself In 30 Days
543-209-5576	832-913-0823
410-281-7635	989-638-2031
978-432-9284	610-438-9312

PHONE NUMBER RECALL TEST—3

Set 1: To Test Yourself Now	Set 2: To Test Yourself in 30 Days
211-398-6592	824-978-6353
818-872-8354	213-614-3976
874-480-6597	315-713-3356
203-762-4536	781-775-3258

Test #5B: Bank Account Numbers

BANK ACCOUNT NUMBER RECALL TEST—1

Set 1: To Test Yourself Now	Set 2: To Test Yourself in 30 Days
1437890652	4682083514

BANK ACCOUNT NUMBER RECALL TEST—2

Set 1: To Test Yourself Now

8935872451

3765598124

Set 2: To Test Yourself in 30 Days

7839822413

9520873365

BANK ACCOUNT NUMBER RECALL TEST—3

Set 1: To Test Yourself Now

1353760972

7649920873

8563200982

Set 2: To Test Yourself in 30 Days

5369837261

4572343987

8379264037

Remembering Faces and Names

How well are you able to remember faces and the names and occupations that go with them? In the following test, you'll see a dozen faces with the information about them. Then, you'll see a set of faces that includes most of the faces you have seen. How well do you remember if you have seen that face and how well do you remember what you know about that person?

Test #6: Faces and Names

Look at the following set of faces for 4 or 5 minutes; then cover it up, and see how much you can remember in the second set. Take this as an immediate or delayed memory test, as you choose.

FACE RECOGNITION TEXT—SET 1

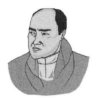

John Henry
CEO

David Aarons
Construction

Sarah Price
Hairdresser

Sam Taylor
Accountant

Danny Williams
Grad Student

Patricia Rodgers
Marketing Manager

Julia Samuels
Airlines Clerk

Dr. Paul Andrews
History Professor

Cindy Allen
Cocktail Waitress

Andrea Collins
Actress

Tim Watkins
Scientist

Wendy Barrows
Editor-in-Chief

FACE RECOGNITION TEST: WHO DO YOU REMEMBER FROM SET 1

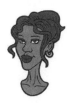 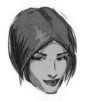 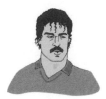

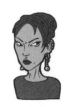 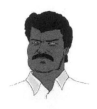 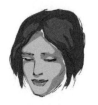 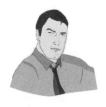

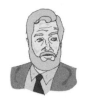 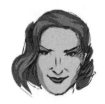 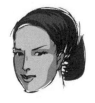 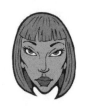

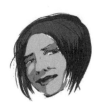 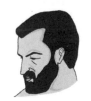 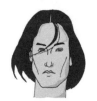 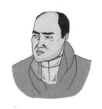

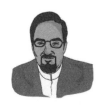 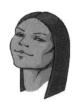 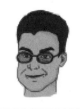 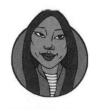

After you fill in as much information as you can for the faces that were in the first test, give yourself 1 point for each correct face recognition, 1 point for the correct name, and 1 point for the correct occupation. Subtract 3 points for each face you incorrectly identify as having been in the first test. Then, try this test again in 30 days, and compare the results. Make sure to write down whether you took this test immediately or after a delay, so that when you repeat the test, you use the same conditions.

Remembering Images

Finally, how well do you remember what you see? To test yourself, the first is a recall test where you draw as much as you can remember. The second is a recognition test, in which you try to remember which images you saw before and what's missing.

Test #7A: Draw It

See how long you can retain a visual image. You can do this as a series of tests or you can draw two, three, or four images at the same time.

Look at each image below for 30 seconds and remember as much as you can. Then, close the book and try to draw it from memory. Next, without looking back at the image or your drawing, do something else for 30 minutes and try to draw it again. Compare your two drawings to the original to see how much you remember. Then, try the same test 30 days later and see how your second set of drawings compare to your first test.

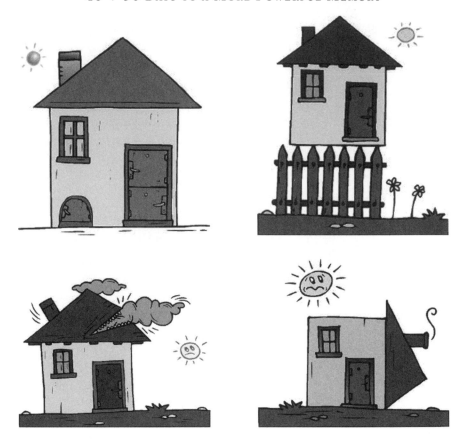

Test #7B: How Much Did You See?

Here's a test where you look at a room or some people doing something and try to remember everything you see there. In fact, you can create your own test for this—just go into a room or observe any group of people, look away, and see how much detail you can remember.

You'll see two similar images for your initial test and your test after 30 days. In each case, look at the image for 1 minute, look away, and write down as many things as you remember. Then, look back at the image and see how many things you have remembered correctly. Score 1 point for each item you correctly remember; deduct 1 point for each item you incorrectly recorded or omitted completely. Then, compare your current and 30 days later scores. While the scenes to look at are slightly different, they are of similar types of scenes for the two time periods.

IN THE OFFICE TEST

Set 1: To Test Yourself Now

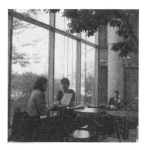

Set 2: To Test Yourself in 30 Days

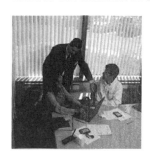

PEOPLE TALKING TEST

Set 1: To Test Yourself Now

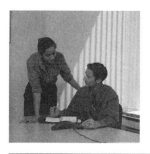

Set 2: To Test Yourself in 30 Days

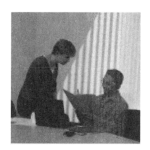

Summing Up

So there you have it, a series of quizzes to test your memory for different types of information—from everyday experiences and observations to words, faces, and images. In fact, just taking the quizzes will help you think more about using your memory, which will contribute to your ability to observe and pay attention and therefore better encode information.

Compare your scores on different quizzes, too, to notice where you have a better memory ability and where you have more difficulty remembering. These differences will help you know where you already excel and where you need to improve in the future. For example, you may be much better at remembering what you observe compared to words or numbers. In turn, these differences may reflect what has been more important to you in your life. But as you concentrate on improving your memory in other areas, you should begin noticing improvements there, too.

4

Creating a Memory Journal

The first step in your 30-day memory plan should be creating a memory journal in which you think about what you remembered, what you didn't remember, notice patterns, and start to pay increased attention to things. This way you create a baseline for where you are now and can track your progress as you move to where you want to be. Since a first step to remembering anything is paying attention (apart from being in good health, getting a good night's sleep so you're alert, and otherwise having your mental equipment tuned up to remember), being attentive to your memory processes will help you focus on remembering more.

So devote your first week to paying attention and upping your awareness of when and how you remember. Besides setting up the journal, described in this chapter, devote this week to some attention exercises to help you pay more attention. Then, as you develop this habit it will carry over into your everyday life.

How to Set Up Your Memory Journal

Set up your journal like a diary or chronology in which you make entries in your diary each day—or even several times a day, as you get ideas related to your memory. You might even consider including the parts of your journal you want to share on a blog. You might even add a section on this to your blog, if you are writing a blog on your own Website or on one of the popular sites for blogging. If you do turn this into a blog or something you share with others, be sure you feel comfortable with others reading what you post. If not, consider just posting those parts of your journal anyone can read and keep the other parts offline. A good way to make the distinction is to keep personal observations and thoughts about yourself in your private offline journal; but if you have any insights about what you can do to improve your memory—which could be useful for anyone else—by all means, post them for all to see.

To make your journal more helpful to you, divide it up into a series of sections, such as listed below, so you have a series of goals for developing your memory, keep track of your successes in remembering different types of information, and note when you experience memory lapses. This way you can notice trends in your ability to remember over time, chart improvements and continuing challenges, and record insights. You can turn this study of your own memory into a chart, with a column for each section.

For example, in your notebook you might have these sections:

1. My overall goal (i.e., what you hope to achieve by the end of 30 days).
2. My goals for today (i.e., the areas of memory improvement you are focusing on now).
3. My memory successes (i.e., specific incidents, experiences, and observations where you enjoyed a notable, outstanding, or unexpected success).
4. My memory lapses (i.e., specific times when you found you weren't able to recall or recognize something at all or where you remembered it incorrectly).
5. Trends and patterns (i.e., types of things you are likely to remember, types of things you find you often forget or remember incorrectly).
6. Memory improvements (i.e., things you find you can remember now that you didn't before).
7. Memory challenges (i.e., things that you are continuing to find especially difficult to remember).

8. Memory insights (i.e., ideas and tips you have gained from your own experiences in trying to remember things or in keeping this journal, plus ideas and tips you have gained from your reading or from others—including talking to people or from radio or TV).

If you turn this into a chart, such as by creating a table in Word or an Excel chart, make each of the above categories a column header.

Then, enter what you feel is most relevant each day, and use these categories to help focus your attention on different aspects of your memory development. You can also use this journal to direct your attention to what you consider the most important areas to work on, so you can better plan and prioritize what to do. In effect, you are using your central executive function, which you read about in Chapter 1, to recall and think about what you have and haven't remembered and decide what to do about this so in the future you remember more.

While the above sections may be a helpful way to divide up the study of your own memory, as an alternative, you can make entries in your journal as a narrative, just keeping those categories in mind so you can incorporate these different topics in your journal as you write.

Most importantly, write in your journal each day if you can, since this way you can better chart your progress and stay focused on what you need to do to improve. Then, too, you will be able to better remember what happened on a day-by-day basis; otherwise, your images and impressions from each successive day will interfere with you remembering what you did the day before. You know the feeling. Someone asks you what you did during your lunch break yesterday, and you very likely have trouble remembering exactly what you did—unless it was something dramatic that cut through the clutter of many thousands of sensory inputs and memories for each day, like observing a fight between two women in the supermarket while you were waiting on line.

If you do skip a day, return to writing your journal as soon as you can and try to recall what happened the day before, along with your thoughts and insights from those experiences.

How to Use the Journal to Improve Your Progress

As you keep notes about what and how you remember in your journal, you can use this to guide what you do.

For example, suppose you note that you have had trouble remembering names at events you attend. That will suggest that you target this area of memory to work on. Or suppose you notice a pattern that you are forgetting things more at certain times of the day. This might suggest that you are more tired and less attentive at this time. You need either to take steps to up your energy (say, getting more sleep or eating an energy snack around that time each day) or to recognize that your memory ability is less sharp at this time, so you find another time to seek to learn something new if you can. In short, use what you learn about your memory powers as you keep your journal to determine what you need to work on or when your memory powers are at a lower ebb.

Conversely, if you note memory successes, take some time to congratulate and reward yourself, which will help to keep you motivated to continue to improve. When you see signs of your success and are rewarded for them, you'll feel even better about what you are doing to increase your memory. For example, say after a history of not remembering the names of most of the people you meet at a business mixer, you consciously work on encoding those names into your memory and find you are better able to make them part of your long-term memory, so you can recall much more—from the details of what they do to what you need to do to follow up with each person. That's great! A terrific achievement! So acknowledge this to yourself and give yourself some reward, such as praising yourself, patting yourself on the back, treating yourself to a coffee latte, or giving yourself a star or blue ribbon. This way you recognize your progress and keep yourself going to the next level of improvement.

A good way to use rewards is to provide a small amount of praise or give a small reward to yourself after a day of good progress. But make the reward even bigger for your achievements for the week.

Then, after 30 days, go all out to reward yourself as well as clearly indicate where you have made your progress. This will show that you have completed 30 days to a better memory successfully—then you can sign on for another 30 days to work on making even more improvements.

Sample Memory Journal

Here's an example of how you might keep a memory journal, based on the first two entries in my own journal. I have used a more narrative approach in keeping this journal, though later on, I frequently broke each daily entry into separate categories, as relevant.

June 28, 2006

Now that I started working on this memory book, I began thinking about paying attention more and thinking of strategies to better memorize things when I prepared for a potential quiz in a Native American class I'm taking. We had about 70 pages of creation stories from different tribes to read, and the stories had a lot of detail. There were also many unfamiliar names, overlapping storylines, and other things making it hard to remember. I began thinking of strategies to make it easier for me to remember and thought about how these might be applicable for others.

- *Read once for the general flow of the story and to enjoy it, though I might bracket major points to review later. Read the story a second time a day or two later to more closely notice detail (like names of key characters, title of the story, what group it refers to) and consciously notice what seems new to me even though I read it before. Then, a day or two later, skim over the story, paying particular attention to what I have underlined.*

- *To remember something even more precisely, I can create a chart with several columns that highlight the major points to remember. For example, for these stories, I might use one column with the name of the story, a second with the major plot line, a third with the names of key characters, and a fourth column to note special themes, lessons, my reactions, and any other thoughts I have about the story.*

I also had a conversation about the class with one of the other students, and she mentioned the difficulty she had remembering the stories. She had read the stories the day after our weekly class, but then she didn't remember what she had read in the class. She didn't even remember having read the stories at all. Based on my own experience of reading each story two or three times—and the last time, the day before the class—her account suggests that it is better to wait until shortly before you have to remember something and allow the time to read it by then; or use the multiple reading and review process I used.

I also recalled how I found it helpful to recall unfamiliar names by not only seeing them visually, but by saying them over in my mind a few times, so I would learn the new information through multiple channels.* Another technique that I found helpful is mentally reviewing what I have read, which also applies to what I have seen or experienced. I just repeat in my mind or use self-talk to tell myself what I want to remember. This way I reinforce my initial information input.

June 29, 2006

As I drove home from school today I began to think of different types of memory exercises, based on noticing things and paying attention. For example, these exercises, which I can do by myself or with others, include:

- *Looking at cards with multiple images where you have to notice what's different.*

- *Observing a scene closely on a card or in reality; then you see the same scene again with something removed. Your job is to notice what's missing. In turn, this exercise might help you pay attention to what's there.*

- *Observing a scene closely as above, except that instead of noticing what's missing, you have to notice and identify what has been added to the scene. Again, another exercise to help in paying attention.*

---

*Though I didn't yet know about the different aspects of the working memory, this would be a good example of improving one's memory by reinforcing it through rehearsal and repetition, and using both imagery through the visuospatial sortbox and words through the phonological loop to drive these names into my long-term memory.

- *Imagining yourself taking a series of pictures of the scene; then you recall as many objects you saw in the scene without looking, and later check your recollection.*

- *Having a mental conversation about what you just did or learned; imagine you are telling yourself or a friend what you just experienced, or imagine you are a teacher instructing your class.*

- *Reflecting on what you have learned or your experience, and consider what it means to you and how you can use this information.*

I also thought about some of the main principles of memory and how they might provide a frame of things to do for the next week. The key ones are:

- *Being well rested and alert (preparatory)*
- *Paying attention—and paying attention to yourself paying attention (so you get the information into your working memory)*
  - *Creating keys to help you pay attention (such as name triggers, mnemonics)*
  - *Recording what you are paying attention to, such as through writing or drawing, to intensify what you are taking in*
  - *Using techniques to make what you have seen or experienced stand out, such as imagining you are a camera taking pictures of a scene; imagining you are a tape recorder recording a conversation*
  - *Using associations with what you have seen/read/experienced, such as images for names, places*
- *Reviewing what you have taken in*
- *Participating in activities to reinforce what you have learned*
- *Prioritizing what you have taken in, so you focus on what is more important*
- *Categorizing and grouping what you have learned, so you can better recall it, since we generally only can take in 7 bits of information (plus or minus 2) together*
- *Sharing what you have observed, read about, or experienced with others, since that intensifies the experience*

- *Keeping a written record, like this memory journal, to notice what you remember more effectively and what you don't, so you can increasingly apply what works in the future*

Similarly, you can develop your own memory journal, where you record what you experienced and what's important to you, along with your ideas on what to do to improve your own memory. You'll see many techniques in this book. But as you keep your journal, you may come up with your own ideas for what you need to better remember and what you might do to increase your memory power.

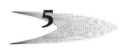

Pay Attention!!!

One reason many people have trouble remembering something is that they don't make a clear picture of what they want to remember, because they don't pay enough attention in the beginning. The crucial first step to remembering anything is to PAY ATTENTION. You have to first take in the information in order to put it in your short-term or working memory and later transfer it to your long-term memory.

Naturally, you can remember all sorts of things without being particularly attentive, as unconsciously you are absorbing information all the time and much of this stays with you, even if you are unaware of it. But, this casual absorption of information can be a hit-or-miss proposition. While you may take in much of this information unconsciously and may later remember things you didn't realize you had even learned, to improve your memory you have to consciously pay attention. This approach is sometimes referred to as being "mindful," as opposed to operating on automatic.

Certainly, you want to continue to keep most everyday processes in your life automatic, since you need to do this to move through everyday life; you can't try to pay close attention to everything you do, since this will slow you down. Yet at the same time, you can become more aware of what you are doing on automatic and you can focus more closely on some usually automatic activities. Then, you can better remember what you want to remember, such as the names of people you meet at a business mixer or trade show.

Learning to Pay Attention

The following exercises are designed to help you pay closer attention to what you do.

Creating a Memory Trigger to Increase Your Ability to Focus

When you're in a situation where it's particularly important to remember something, you can remind yourself to pay close attention by using a "memory trigger." This trigger can be almost any type of gesture or physical sign—such as bringing your thumb and forefinger together, clasping your hands so your thumbs and index finger create a spire, or raising your thumb. Or you could use a mental statement to remind yourself to pay attention. Whatever signal you choose, it's designed to remind you that it's now time to be especially alert and listen or watch closely, so you'll remember all you can. If you already have a signal you like, use that, or use the following exercise to create this trigger.

> Get relaxed, perhaps close your eyes. Then, ask yourself this question: "What mental trigger would I like to use to remind myself to pay attention?" Notice what comes into your mind. It may be a gesture, a physical movement, a mental image, or a word or phrase you say to yourself. Choose that as your trigger.
>
> Now, to give power to this trigger, make the gesture or movement or let this image or word appear in your mind. Then, as you make this gesture or observe the image or word, repeatedly use this gesture for a minute or two, and as you do, say to yourself with increasing intensity: "I will pay attention now. I will be very alert and aware, and I will lock this information in my memory so I can recall it later." This process of using the gesture and paying attention will associate the act of paying attention with the gesture.
>
> Later (either the same day or the following day if you are beginning this exercise at night), practice using this trigger in some real-life situations. Find three or more times when you are especially interested in

remembering something, and use your trigger to make yourself more alert. For example, when you see something you would especially like to remember (such as someone on the street, a car on the road, etc.), use your trigger to remind you to pay attention to it. Afterwards, when whatever you have seen is gone, replay it mentally in as much detail as possible to illustrate how much you can remember when you really pay attention.

Initially, to reinforce the association with the sign you have created, as you make this gesture, repeat the same words to yourself as in your concentration exercises: "I will pay attention now. I will be very alert and aware, and I will lock this information in my memory so I can recall it later." Then, look or listen attentively to whatever it is you want to remember.

Repeat both the meditation and the real-life practice for a week to condition yourself to associate the action you want to perform (paying attention) with the trigger (raising your thumb, etc.). Once this association is locked in, continue to use the trigger in real life. As long as you continue to regularly use the trigger, you don't need to continue practicing the exercise, since each time you use the trigger, your attention will be on high alert.

Then, any time you are in an important situation where you want to pay especially careful attention (such as a staff meeting or a cocktail party with prospective clients), use your trigger, and you'll become more attentive and alert.

Using a Physical Trigger or Motion to Keep Your Attention Focused

To keep yourself from drifting off while you are listening to something or to keep your mind from wandering while you are observing or experiencing something, you can use the trigger you have created or any gesture or physical signal to remind yourself to pay attention to what you are hearing or seeing.

For example, every 20 or 30 seconds, click your fingers softly, move a toe, or move another part of your body as a reminder. Once you decide on the trigger, practice this signal to make the association with paying attention by repeatedly making this gesture and after that focus your attention on something. Then, that gesture or motion will become your trigger to pay attention.

After a while, should your attention drift away, simply repeat the trigger to bring you back to attention again.

Using Clear Memory Pictures or Recordings to Improve Your Memory

Another way to pay closer attention is to make a sharp mental picture or recording of the person, place, or event you want to remember. This process will also help you with the second phase of the memory retention process, where you encode this information using visual imagery or sounds. But this first phase is what picks up the information in the first place, much like using a camera or a cassette.

A major factor in poor remembering is that often we don't make this picture or recording very well. As a result, we may think we remember what we have seen, but we don't. Courtroom witnesses, for example, often recall an event inaccurately, although they may be positive they are correct. Accordingly, before you can recall or recognize something properly in the retrieval stage of the process, you first must have a clear impression of it.

One way to do this, once you are paying careful attention, is to think of yourself as a camera or cassette recorder, taking in completely accurate pictures or recordings of what you are experiencing. As you observe and listen, make your impressions like pictures or tape recordings in your mind.

It takes practice to develop this ability, and the following exercises are designed to help you do this. At first, use these exercises to get a sense of how well you already remember what you see. Then, as you practice, you'll find you can remember more and more details.

The underlying principle of these exercises is to observe some object, person, event, or setting to take a picture, or listen to a conversation or other sounds around you. Then, turn away from what you are observing or stop listening, and recall what you can. Perhaps write down what you recall. Finally, look back and ask yourself: "How much did I remember? What did I forget? What did I recall that wasn't there?"

At first, you may be surprised at how bad an observer or listener you are. But as you practice, you'll improve—and your skill at remembering will carry over into other situations, because you'll automatically start making more accurate memory pictures or recordings in your mind.

An ideal way to use these techniques is with a mental awareness trigger. Whenever you use that trigger, you will immediately imagine yourself as a camera or recorder and indelibly impress that scene on your mind for later recall.

The next three exercises are designed to give you some practice in perceiving like a camera or cassette recorder in a private controlled setting. The fourth exercise is one you can use in any situation to perceive more effectively.

Looking at Things More Accurately

This exercise will help increase your powers of observation.

> *Look at a scene in front of you that has a lot of different things in it. These can be different objects, people who are mostly stationery (i.e., sitting down, not a bustling crowd), scenery, etc. Or use a picture of such a scene. Then, stare at this scene for about a minute, and as you do, imagine you are taking a picture of it, as if your mind is a camera taking a snapshot. As you do so, notice as many things about the scene as you can. Pay attention to forms, colors, the number of objects or people there, the relationship between things, etc.*
>
> *Then, look away from that scene, and try to recreate it as accurately as possible in your mind's eye. As when you really looked at the scene, notice the forms, colors, number of objects or people, and the relationship between things.*
>
> *Next, to check your accuracy, without looking back, write down a list of what you saw in as much detail as possible.*
>
> *Finally, rate your accuracy and your completeness by rating your observations. To score your level of accuracy, designate each accurate observation with a +2. Score each inaccurate observation with a −1. Score each invented observation with a −2. Then, tally up your score and note the result. To score your level of completeness, estimate the total number of observations you think were possible in the scene and divide by the number of observations you made, to get your completeness score. As you*

continue to practice with this exercise, you'll find your score for both accuracy and completeness should go up.

Listening to What You Hear

This exercise will help you become more aware of what you hear and help you listen more completely and correctly.

Tape a short segment of conversation or some sounds on a tape cassette. You can record this from an ongoing conversation, from a television or radio program, or from ambient sounds on the street around you. Tape for 2 to 3 minutes.

Then, while you are taping or later when you play back the recording, concentrate on listening as intently and carefully as possible. Imagine you are a tape recorder that is recording every bit of conversation clearly and accurately. Either way, as you are taping or playing back the recording, really listen. Perhaps form images in your mind as you do.

At the end of the recording, try to recall the conversation or sounds in as much detail as possible. Perhaps imagine yourself as a tape recorder playing this back. Additionally, try to remember what you heard in sequence as best you can.

To check your accuracy, write down a list of what you heard in as much detail as possible. You needn't write everything down word for word, but write down enough to indicate the gist of each thought or statement. Then, play back the tape, and review how complete and accurate you were.

Finally, rate your accuracy and completeness by rating your recall of the conversation. To score your level of accuracy, designate each accurate recollection with a +2. Score each inaccurate recollection with a −1. Score each invented recollection with a −2. Then, tally up your score and note the result. To score your level of completeness, estimate the total number of recollections you think were possible in what you heard and divide by the number of recollections you made, to get your completeness score. Give yourself 10 bonus points if you got everything in sequence; 5 bonus points if you got most things in sequence. Finally, total and divide this result by your estimated number of total sounds, statements, or phrases for your percentage rating.

As you continue to practice with this exercise, you'll find your score for both accuracy and completeness should go up.

Seeing Like a Camera; Listening Like a Cassette Recorder

This exercise will help you observe or listen more accurately and completely in everyday situations.

You can use this technique wherever you are—it's especially ideal for parties, business networking meetings, and other important occasions where you want to be sure to remember things accurately. Also, you can use this technique to practice and sharpen your skills when you're waiting in line, traveling in a bus, in a theater lobby at intermission, and in places where you are waiting for something to happen.

Simply imagine you are a camera and snap a picture of what you see. Or imagine you are a cassette recorder picking up a conversation. Or be a sound film camera and pick up both.

Afterwards, turn away or close your eyes if convenient, and for a few seconds, focus on what you have just seen or heard. If you have taken a picture, visualize it intently in your mind's eye and concentrate. What objects or people do you see? What colors or details do you notice? What furniture is in the room? What are the people wearing?

Then, look at the scene and compare your picture with what you see now. What did you leave out? What did you add that wasn't there? What details did you observe incorrectly? The more you do this, the more complete and accurate your picture will be.

If you have tried to listen like a cassette recorder, replay what you have heard in your mind. What did people say? What sounds did you hear around you? You won't be able to actually hear these conversations or sounds again, but you can get a sense of how much detail you were able to pick up. The more you practice, the more fully you will hear.

If you have imagined yourself as a sound film camera, review both the pictures and sounds.

Experiencing an Object

This exercise will help you become more aware of what you see and help you perceive more completely and correctly.

Place a common object or group of objects in front of you (such as a collection of objects from your desk, a painting on your wall, an advertisement or picture from a magazine, a flower arrangement in a vase). Stare at the object or group of objects for about a minute, and notice as many things about it as you can, such as its form, texture, color, design, pattern, and so on. Be aware of how many objects there are, and catalog the names of all the objects in your mind.

Then, remove the object, or groups of objects, so it is out of sight, but continue looking at the spot where it was, and imagine the object(s) as still there. Try to recreate what you saw with as much detail as you can.

To check your accuracy, write down a list of what you saw. Then, look at what you observed again and see how accurate you were.

To chart your progress each time, score the total number of observations you think were possible (this will vary with each observer), and score each of your accurate observations with a +2. Score each of your inaccurate observations with a −1, and your invented observations with a −2. Finally, total and divide by your estimated number of total observations for your percentage rating.

As you continue to practice with this exercise, you'll find your rating will go up.

More Tips for Paying Attention

Using Note Taking to Stay Focused

Another way to better pay attention, as well as better encode material later, since you are using more sensory input channels, is to take notes in situations where it is appropriate to do so (such as when you are listening to a lecture in class, to a speech, or to a discussion at a meeting). Even if you never look at the notes later, just the process of taking the notes will keep you more mentally alert as you listen and observe more attentively. Plus the note taking will reinforce what you hear, since you will take in the information visually (what you write down) and kinetically (the physical process of writing down what you hear).

The way to take good notes is to write down key points the person is making. The act of writing will focus your attention so you absorb more information. Take detailed notes if that helps you better understand and think about what you are hearing. Alternatively, if a lot of writing interferes with listening to what is coming next, just write down main phrases and concepts. The key is to write something to keep you alert and focused.

That's what Alison, a college student, discovered. Initially, she found it hard to listen to lectures, because she would grow restless and her mind would drift, and she would begin thinking about all sorts of things other than the lecture—what happened the night before, the patterns of sunlight on the leaves outside, her plans for tomorrow. Then, suddenly, she would realize she had drifted off and pull herself back, but by then she had missed several minutes of lecture, and after a few minutes, she would drift off again.

But finally, she overcame the problem by taking notes as quickly as she could, which focused her mind on the lecture by forcing her to pay attention, even though she might not need all the information. Later, she could decide what information was useful. As a result, she did better in her classes, because she remembered more. And later, she transferred her skill at note taking to pay attention into the business world. There, taking comprehensive notes at meetings not only helped her stay focused but provided a detailed record she could use in writing up reports and action memos based on the meetings.

Listening Proactively

Another way to stay attentive, as well as make a memory more vivid when you encode it, is to use proactive listening where you react to and comment mentally on what you are hearing. You can think about what you are hearing, because we think several times faster than people speak. For example, when you listen to a lecture or a conversation, the person talks at about one third or one quarter the rate at which you can think. So you can use that additional time to actively reflect on what that person is saying—say, by responding with a mental commentary. That time lag between speaking and thinking also allows you to take detailed notes at a lecture while still listening to the speaker—you are in effect writing in between the spaces. Both the mental commentary and the process of note taking are ways to help you stay attentive.

This proactive listening—actively thinking while you listen—will force you to pay more attention since you are processing and responding to this material, not just taking it in.

For example, say you are listening to a speech. You might ask yourself questions like: What is the speaker's main point here? What do I think about it? Do I agree or disagree?

Obviously, you don't want to let this technique cause you to get so caught up in your questions and commentary that you stop listening to something and go off on a mental tangent. Thus, keep your mental questions or comments short, so you can quickly return back to what the person is saying. In short, you are engaging in a mental dialogue with the person you are listening to, so you are listening more proactively, but not slipping into a mental monologue where you get so caught up in your own thoughts that you tune the speaker out.

While this mental dialogue process is ideal when you are a passive listener, you can also use it when you are having an extended conversation with someone, particularly if it turns to a serious discussion. The technique is ideal to keep you focused and more attentive to what the person is saying.

Initially, you have to remind yourself to use this process, say by using a trigger. But after a while it will become second nature, so you can listen proactively whenever you want. This technique can also work in an extended conversation you are having with a friend or colleague, to keep you focused and more attentive to what the person is saying.

Observing Proactively

Just as listening attentively and proactively will help you remember more, so will observing proactively. The process is similar to what you do when you listen this way.

In this case, as you observe something, you don't only passively receive this information, but you actively respond to it as you receive it. For example, as you look at something, reflect on what you are seeing. Talk to yourself about what you are seeing and what you think and feel about it. Perhaps compare what you are seeing now to something else you have seen that looks the same or looks different (such as you might do in seeing a painting in an art gallery, comparing the landscape in one country to the landscape in another).

Increasing Your Ability to Maintain Interest

If you find your interest flagging as you are trying to pay attention, concentrate, or make connections, try taking a quick mental break or injecting a quick dose of humor to boost your energy to stay focused and attentive. The process is a little like the runner who stops for a moment on the track for a quick energy drink to get that push to go on. Likewise, you may need a quick infusion of mental energy to stay on track.

Here are a few suggestions for quick mental energy breaks—and you can think of others yourself:

1. Tell yourself "Time Out," and glance around for a few seconds taking mental pictures, as you imagine yourself getting a charge of energy from each picture. When you focus back on your task, imagine that this renewed energy charge is spreading through you, giving you more and more energy for what you are doing.

2. As you look at a person who is talking, think of a funny statement, image, or joke that might fit that person. Then, after a few seconds of comic relief, feel energized and ready to go on again in a more serious vein.

3. Do a quick energy recharging exercise. Think of an image of power and energy (such as a picture of a professional athlete, rocket, or flashing neon sign saying "Energy"), and as you do, say an energy-increasing affirmation to yourself, such as: "I am feeling energized . . . I am feeling energized . . . I feel more power and energy than ever . . . I feel more power and energy than ever."

Then, after your mental energy break, return feeling recharged and ready to go again.

Prepare Yourself to Pay Attention

Now try putting these techniques for paying attention into practice. Before you go to a meeting, have a conversation with someone, or any other event, remind yourself that you will actively react in your mind to what is said, and if you expect to take notes, remind yourself that you will take these in as much detail as possible. Also, remind yourself that you will actively react in your mind to what the person is saying and what you are writing. If you go to view something (such as in an art gallery or on a sightseeing trip), remind yourself that you will actively think about what you are seeing and compare and contrast it with other things.

In short, before you do something where you want to better focus, concentrate, and learn more, remind yourself to approach the experience in an active information-receiving and -perceiving mode. Then you will actively react to what you are seeing, and you may incorporate this information in another sensory channel, as well.

6

Improving Your Health and Your Memory

Your health and general well-being play a major role in how well your memory works, so improving them will also improve your ability to remember. Again and again, researchers have found a strong correlation between good health, eating a healthy diet with good nutrition, getting sufficient sleep, exercising your body, being in a good emotional state and mood, and staying away from alcohol and drugs, smoking (tobacco *and* marijuana), and toxic chemicals. So I want to touch briefly on these basics here, though the focus in this book is on the mental and perceptual techniques you can use for memory improvement.

Consider being in good health, eating and sleeping well, getting sufficient exercise, and being in a good mood the foundations of your memory house. Most of this book deals with building that dream house; but if you don't have a strong foundation on which to build, the whole house will come down.

While this chapter provides a basic overview for maintaining a strong foundation or strengthening it, for more details look at books that deal specifically with these topics. When it comes to making more specific choices for yourself, consult a professional, such as a nutritionist, psychologist, or medical professional.

Sleep on It

Getting enough sleep is critical for having a good memory, because if you are tired, your memory won't work as well. You have probably experienced this yourself—you are trying to pay attention and absorb new information, and you keep drifting off. Even if you are able to force yourself to pay attention, you won't be able to encode what you learn as well. And if you try to retrieve information, your lack of alertness will slow you down. It's like trying to drive a run-down car that keeps overheating or slowing down.

Aside from needing your sleep to stay alert, researchers have also found that the mind goes through certain mental processes at night while you are sleeping and dreaming that help to solidify memories in your mind. How? According to researchers, as described by Karen Markowitz and Eric Jensen in *The Great Memory Book,* the more you learn during the day, you more you are likely to dream or need to dream. Dreaming occurs when you go through a period of rapid eye-movement, referred to as REM sleep, which takes up about 25 percent of your overall sleep period. Typically this occurs for about two hours a night, broken up into four or five 20- to 30-minute periods. During this time, the cerebral cortex, which plays a critical role in long-term memory processing, is especially active, and researchers believe that when you sleep, this part of the brain plays a role in learning consolidation.[1]

In other words, it's like sending what you have learned for the day—what you have newly encoded into a memory—to a storage area to be turned into a bound copy for your memory archive. If you've gotten sufficient sleep, the production process will go well, and your memory will be bound into your long-term memory for easy retrieval. But if you haven't slept well, the process may break down, so you won't be able to get that memory transferred into long-term memory properly or there will be flaws in that stored memory.

Thus, besides setting aside sufficient time for sleep (generally 7–8 hours, though some people find that they can do well with only 5–6 hours of sleep), take steps to ensure you have a good night's sleep. Some tips[2] suggested by John B. Arden, the Director of Training for Psychology at the Kaiser Permanente Medical Centers in Northern California,[3] include:

- Don't drink a large amount of liquids throughout the evening, since this may wake you up during the night to go to the bathroom.

- Don't try too hard to fall asleep, since you will release neurotransmitters, such as epinephrine and norepinephrine, which activate various body systems, such as your heart rate, blood pressure, and muscle tension. If you have difficulty falling asleep, try getting up for awhile, then try again when you feel sleepy.

- Don't work under a strong light late at night, since this will trick your brain into thinking it's daytime.

- Take care of any planning you need to do for the next day before you go to bed, so you are not thinking about what you need to do as you try to fall asleep. If you do suddenly remember something, jot it down on a bedside notepad so you don't have to worry about whether you will remember.

- If you need help falling asleep or going back to sleep if you wake up, try using a relaxation exercise, which are described in Chapter 7.

- Shut out any noise that bothers you with earplugs.

- Avoid eating foods that will increase your energy before going to bed, such as foods with high sugar or salt content or high protein, though a light snack with complex carbohydrates is fine, such as granola or a bowl of multi-grain cereal.

- Don't take naps during the day, since this may make it harder for you to feel sleepy and fall asleep at night.

Arden also suggests only using your bed for sleeping and sex, and not doing everyday activities like eating, watching television, balancing your checkbook, or having a discussion with your spouse.[4] This way you reinforce the association between bed and sleep, though many people, myself included, can readily do other activities in their beds without interfering with their sleep patterns. In addition, you might close the door to the room where you are sleeping, if this helps you feel more contained and focused on sleeping.

Finally, while numerous entrepreneurs and promoters have made big bucks selling records and tapes that you can listen to in order to learn while you sleep, it doesn't work. According to author Douglas J. Herrmann, author of *Super Memory*, people do not learn while they are asleep. If you play a tape and learn something from it, you are actually remembering what you heard while you are awake—say while you are falling asleep or if you wake up during the night. But while you are really asleep you don't learn anything.[5] Some researchers have found, however, that if you go to sleep right after learning something, you will remember more than if you engage in other activities between learning and going to bed. Herrmann additionally suggests that you "avoid eating and drinking late at night, avoid thinking about your troubles prior to bedtime, and go to bed at approximately the same time every night."[6]

You Are What You Eat

Your diet has a major impact on your memory, too, so if you eat a healthy diet, you will remember more. There is general agreement on the basics of what constitutes a healthy diet—eating a good mix of protein, carbohydrates, good fats, fiber, and vitamins and minerals. Especially good foods include fresh fruits, vegetables, whole grains, and proteins.

A key reason that eating well will help you remember, according to numerous nutritionists and authors, is that the neurotransmitters that enable one cell to communicate with another require a great deal of energy to function[7]—even more so than other organs in your body. The brain uses 20 percent of your body's oxygen even though it takes up only 2 percent of your whole body weight. It continually has to be supplied by fuel from oxygen and your blood sugar (also called glucose), supplied by your bloodstream, since the brain has no capacity to store energy. As a result, when the glucose level in your blood drops down too far, your brain will draw that energy it needs from other organs, leading you to feel "foggy-headed"; you may find it difficult to concentrate or worse, such as experiencing amnesia and having less ability to think and reason.[8]

Then, too, your brain needs antioxidants, since it is susceptible to oxidation, so you need foods that provide this, such as foods that have a high level of vitamin C, vitamin E, carotenoids, and selenium.[9] In addition, good sources of brain nutrition include the omega-3 fatty acids, B vitamins, and certain minerals. [10]

Thus, maintaining a healthy diet is critical—another building block in the foundation of having a good memory. So if you are not already eating well, take steps to improve your diet.

Eating a Healthy Diet

Here are some general suggestions[11]; for more details, look at books on nutrition, visit a nutritionist, or ask your doctor for advice on what to eat.

- Eat plenty of fruits and vegetables, since these are a good source of antioxidants.
- Eat breads made with complex grains, such as rye and whole wheat, rather than processed white flour.
- Eat less of or avoid red meat, egg yolks, butter, or margarine.
- Reduce the amount of salt you use.
- Reduce the fats you eat by eating low-fat foods, such as low-fat milk and cheese and ice cream. In particular, reduce the saturated fats you eat, that is, those found in butter, coconut oil, egg yolks, meats, and whole meat.
- Reduce the fried food you eat, because these have trans fatty acid—the fats that occur when you heat vegetable oils to a high temperature.
- Look for foods with unsaturated fats, which come in two types: monounsaturated and polyunsaturated. The first type includes several types of oil: olive oil, canola oil, and peanut oil. The second type is even better for you and includes certain vegetable oils, seeds, nuts, and cold-water fish (such as albacore tuna, haddock, mackerel, and salmon).[12]
- Try to eat a balanced meal, which includes a fruit and vegetable, protein, and complex carbohydrate.
- Drink plenty of water.

More specifically, some of the recommendations on good foods to eat include the following from David Thomas, one of the 15 International Grandmasters of Memory and a World Memory Championship medalist in the United States, who broke an 18-year record in *The Guinness Book of Records* for reciting pi to 22,500 digits from memory.[13]

GOOD SOURCES OF NUTRIENTS

Type of Nutrient	Food Sources
Antioxidants, which include vitamin C, vitamin E, selenium, and carotenoids	Citrus fruits, broccoli, peppers, carrots, sweet potatoes, kale, spinach, seafood, grains, brazil nuts, soybeans, vegetable oils
Omega-3 fatty acids	Oily fish, such as sardines, salmon, mackerel, tuna, herring, and anchovies; olive oil
B vitamins, which include B_1, B_2, B_3, B_6, and B_{12}	Poultry, fish, milk, cereal, nuts, whole grains, beans, leafy green vegetables
Minerals, notably boron, magnesium, and zinc	Apples, pears, beans, peas, whole wheat, nuts, dark turkey meat, shellfish

Foods with certain amino acids that manufacture neurotransmitters are ideal, most notably L-glutamine, found in foods like avocados, eggs, peaches, granola, and peas; L-tryptophan, found in foods like almonds, cottage cheese, milk, soybeans, and turkey; and L-phenylalanine, found in foods like chicken, lima beans, milk, peanuts, soybeans, and yogurt.[14]

There are also certain vitamins and minerals that contribute to building your brain, and therefore your memory. These include the following[15]:

- Vitamin A, which is a good antioxidant
- The B vitamins, especially B_1 (thiamine), B_3 (niacin), and B_{12} (cyanocobalamin), which are catalysts for many chemical reactions in your brain

- Vitamin C, which is also a good antioxidant and helps your brain use protein to make neurotransmitters
- Vitamin E, which helps to supply oxygen to your muscles and brain; it's also considered one of the most beneficial antioxidants on the market, acting against the toxic byproducts called free radicals that are deposited in the brain by the blood[16]
- The big three minerals—boron, zinc, and magnesium—plus manganese, iron, calcium, copper, and selenium

Then, too, foods with certain other brain-cell fats, called phospholipids, contribute to your brain processing and power, too. Phophatidyl choline increases the amount of acetylcholine in the brain, which helps to transmit messages from one nerve cell to another. And phosphatidyl serine promotes metabolism and increases the flexibility of cell membranes as they stiffen due to the aging process.[17]

By contrast, the foods to eat less of, because they have high levels of sugar or salt, include[18]:

- Candy, cookies, and cake
- Salted pork rinds, corn chips, salted pretzels, and salted crackers
- Sugary and/or caffeinated sodas

In moderate amounts, coffee can make you more alert, since caffeine is a stimulant that increases the blood flow to the brain. It also increases the level of the neurotransmitters dopamine and norepinephrine, helping you feel more charged up. But if you take too much, it can interfere with your ability to concentrate and use your memory effectively. Why? Because caffeine raises your adrenaline level and increases your feelings of stress, and you may even experience tension headaches and get withdrawal headaches when you come down from a caffeine high.[19]

There are some food additives in processed foods that are best to avoid if you can, notably aspartame and monosodium glutamate (MSG). While aspartame is commonly used as a substitute for sugar such as in NutraSweet—a noble goal, since sugar is itself a memory detractor—it has its own problems. According to psychologist John B. Arden, when you consume a lot of aspartame, the danger is that you may overexcite and thereby damage your brain neurons.[20] So if you can, reduce your consumption of sweet foods and drinks.

As for MSG, which is commonly found in snack chips, seasonings, and soups, it can overexcite your neurons too by stimulating the neurotransmitter glutamate; some neurons can even become exhausted and die as a result.[21] So go easy on the MSG, though it can be hard to avoid in today's processed food age.

In short, you're doing well if you eat a balanced diet that is high in fresh vegetables and fruit, complex carbohydrates, protein from foods with the good fats, and plenty of water and fruit or vegetable juices. Here's a chart of brain food recommendations you might use, suggested by Karen Markowitz and Eric Jensen in *The Great Memory Book*.[22]

GOOD FOODS TO EAT TO NOURISH YOUR BRAIN

Food Category	Types of Food
Fresh vegetables	Leafy greens, broccoli, peas, carrots, potatoes
Fresh fruits	Bananas, avocados, blueberries, oranges, strawberries, tomatoes
Good proteins	Tuna, salmon, yogurt, eggs, dark turkey, organ meats, sardines, anchovies, mackerel, shellfish, soybeans
Carbohydrates	Whole grains, beans, sunflower seeds, nuts
Beverages	Pure water, green tea, fruit juice

Markowitz and Jensen also have put together a list of the top 10 "super-memory foods," along with the different types of vitamins and minerals they contain that are good for your brain.[23] I've combined these together into a handy table, where you will see the recommended vitamins and minerals mentioned again and again.

THE TOP 10 SUPER-MEMORY FOODS[24]

Type of Food	Nutrients
Fish (especially cold-water fish, such as trout, salmon, tuna, herring, mackerel, and sardines)	Lecithin (choline), phenylalanine, ribonucleic acid, tyrosine, DMAE, vitamin B_6, niacin/B_3, copper, protein, zinc, omega-3 fatty acids (DHA), vitamin B_{12}
Eggs	Phenylalanine, lecithin (choline), vitamin B_6, vitamin E
Soybeans	Lecithin (choline), glutamic acid, phenylalanine, vitamin E, iron, zinc, protein, vitamin B_6
Lean beef	Phenylalanine, lecithin (choline), tyrosine, glutamic acid, iron, zinc
Chicken livers	Tyrosine, vitamin A, vitamin B_1, vitamin B_6, vitamin B_{12}, protein, iron
Whole wheat	Lecithin (choline), glutamic acid, vitamin B_6, magnesium, vitamin E, vitamin B_1
Chicken	Phenylalanine, vitamin B_6, niacin/B_3, protein
Bananas	Tyrosine, magnesium, potassium, vitamin B_6
Low-fat dairy products	Phenylalanine, tyrosine, glutamine, protein, ALC, vitamin B_{12}
Avocados	Tyrosine, magnesium

Plus add in other foods that are high in the essentials of good nutrition in each of these categories. As you eat to improve your memory, you're also improving your health and weight generally, for improving your health and memory go together. As one improves, so does the other.

Using Herbs, Supplements, and Memory-Enhancing Medications

You'll see a number of memory-improvement programs suggesting you take different types of herbs or supplements to increase your brain power. Some suggest different types of prescription drugs to enhance memory, too. How well do they work? In general, they mainly contribute to your overall health and level of brain functioning, rather than being the magic key to a better memory, according to Dr. Douglas J. Mason, a Florida neuropsychologist called "The Memory Doctor," who specializes in treating people with brain injuries and other cognitive disorders.[25]

So if you aren't getting certain nutrients in your diet, supplements can certainly be a way to replace these, though ideally you should get as much as possible from what you eat. Supplements might be a good way to get the essential vitamins associated with improved mental processing mentioned above—such as vitamins A, B_1, B_2, B_3, B_6, B_{12}, C, and E—and to get the minerals that contribute, such as boron, zinc, and magnesium, plus manganese, iron, calcium, copper, and selenium.

Some of the other supplements that are commonly recommended[26] are discussed below. (However, check with a nutritionist or your doctor before taking any of these supplements, since different supplements may be more appropriate for different people and dosages can vary.)

- Ginkgo baloba, which comes from the oldest living tree humans know about, has been found to improve memory functioning in healthy adults. It improves the circulation, which brings more nutrients and oxygen to the brain, so the brain operates more effectively. It also has been found to increase the brain's supply of glucose and its ability to use it; this increases brain power because glucose is the brain's main source of fuel and energy.

- DHEA (dehydroepiandrosterone), a hormone produced by the adrenal glands, has been shown to improve memory, and especially long-term memory, in animals. It does this by producing a key brain cell messenger and encouraging the growth of synapses that send signals between cells. While humans produce plenty of this hormone when younger, with age the production level goes down, so a supplement may be helpful for older adults, though its effectiveness and safety are still under review.

- Piracetam, one of the most well-known supplements for improving cognitive functioning, has been widely used for the past two decades. Among other things, it increases cellular communication between the left and right brain hemispheres and increases the metabolism and energy level of the neurons. It has been marketed under various trade names, including Nootropyl and Nootropil.

- DMAE (dimethylaminoethanol), which is more commonly known as "deanol" or the trade name Deaner, has been found to increase the production of acetylcholine, the main neurotransmitter used to facilitate learning and memory.

- Cholinesterase inhibitors, which block the breakdown of acetylcholine, are prescribed by many medical practitioners to slow down memory deterioration. Though they don't stop or cure memory problems, they do reduce some memory problems by increasing the amount of acetylcholine in the brain. Among the major drugs in this category are tacrine, also known as Cognex; donepezil, also known as Aricept; rivastigmine, also known as Exelon; and galantamine, also known as Galantamine.[27] The bottom line is that you probably don't need these if you have no serious memory problems, but if you are starting to have some problems, they might help stop further deterioration.

Besides the supplements and drugs already mentioned, according to Karen Markowitz and Eric Jensen of the Brain Store, more than 100 brain agents, called "nootropics," are under development around the world,[28] which shows the great interest in this area. While many of these are being developed to treat Alzheimer's disease and other conditions causing a loss of memory with aging, many also contribute to a better memory for healthy individuals of all ages.

At the same time, some drugs that you may be taking for some other condition can interfere with your memory. If you notice any loss of memory, be sure to bring this up with your doctor—and be sure to bring along a complete list of the medications you are taking. Your doctor may be able to change the medication or the dosage. These potentially problematic drugs are really quite extensive and include medications for blood pressure, psychiatric and neurological conditions, stomach problems, colds and allergies, heart disease, PIN (or dysplasia) sleeping problems, depression, and diabetes, as well as antibiotics, antipsychotics, and just about any other condition you might take a drug for.[29]

According to Dr. Aaron P. Nelson, author of the *Harvard Medical School Guide to Achieving Optimal Memory*, if you find your memory declining after you start a new medication, there could be a connection. As Nelson points out, there are a wide range of prescription drugs for numerous conditions that can impair your memory, particularly any medication that makes you drowsy, since it makes it hard to concentrate. Among these are tranquilizers, sleeping pills, and certain antihistamines. Also, any anticholinergic agents and many antidepressants can interfere with memory because they block the activity of acetylcholine, one of the neurotransmitters that contributes to transfer of messages from cell to cell. Then, too, if you take narcotic painkillers, such as morphine, beta-blockers for hypertension, or sleeping pills, those often interfere with memory as well.

How do you know if you have a problem from a drug you are taking? You should know fairly quickly, since the effects generally occur within days or weeks of starting a new medication. In some cases, the side effects may disappear as your body adjusts to the medication, but not always, so as long as you take the drug the side effects will continue. Thus, it's important to notify your doctor as soon as you notice any memory difficulties, so he or she can change the dosage or switch you to another medication. List any medications you are currently taking regularly, so your doctor can assess whether there are any drug interactions that are contributing to the problem.[30]

In summary, if you want to go the brain booster route, there is a growing cornucopia of pills and products you can take, though I'm emphasizing improving your memory the natural way—through maintaining a good foundation with good health, nutrition, and sleeping patterns, and using a variety of mind power techniques to improve your memory.

Reducing or Avoiding Alcohol, Marijuana, Other Drugs, and Smoking

While alcohol, marijuana, and assorted recreational drugs may help you relax and spark up your leisure with others, these can also detract from your memory, particularly when you are a regular user. The reason is that the effects of these drugs interfere with your ability to concentrate and remember.

Alcohol can be especially dangerous, and its use is full of myths, such as that it can help you feel less stress and anxiety, can pull you out of a depression, and helps you get to sleep. According to psychologist John B. Arden, alcohol actually makes it more difficult to deal with stress, can make you feel depressed after your last drink, lead you to feel anxious or even have panic attacks, and is well known to cause sleep problems.[31] Researchers have also found that regular alcohol drinkers show poorer performance on memory tests of perception, have poorer short-term memory, and have a reduced ability to learn abstract ideas and to think conceptually. Plus if you are a heavy drinker, you might develop Korsakoff's syndrome, a serious memory disorder in which you suffer major damage to your hippocampus, which connects the right and left brain, have serious working and long-term memory loss, and may even become psychotic.[32] So to the caution "Don't Drink and Drive," you might add: "Don't Drink and Trust Your Memory."

As for marijuana, it may have some good medical effects, make food taste better, and improve your appetite, but it also has a number of negative effects on your memory. As anyone who has used marijuana can tell you, it can lead you to have difficulty paying attention and holding information in your short-term or working memory. In addition, regular marijuana smokers commonly have trouble maintaining clear thoughts and can have fuzzy disorganized memories. In addition, regular users often tend to lack motivation and initiative, and have been noted to become mildly depressed, which lowers your ability to remember, too. [33]

As for other recreational drugs, like Ecstasy, speed, and LSD, these can also interfere with your memory. Essentially, anything that changes your perception or speeds you up will disrupt your memory processing activities in your brain, and regular use can make these changes permanent.

Finally, quit smoking cigarettes if you can. Ironically, the nicotine in a cigarette is a stimulant that can initially help you concentrate and remember, since nicotine helps boost acetylocholine, one of the neurotransmitters that helps memory and learning. But the downside is that smoking leads to serious memory problems (apart from the many other health problems associated with smoking, such as increasing your chances of cancer and emphysema). For example, it can restrict and interrupt blood flow that can lead to strokes resulting in severe memory loss.[34] So don't let your memory go up in smoke due to smoking. Stop smoking now.

Exercise, Exercise, Exercise

Getting plenty of exercise is still another way to help your memory, as well as improve your health and well-being generally. Some of the positives of exercising are described below:

- It helps the brain gain the nutrients it needs and makes you more alert by increasing your metabolism and breathing rate—and your energy.

- It helps to keep the organ systems that support your brain, such as your lungs, heart, and arteries, healthy.

- It stimulates the nerve growth factor (NGF) in your brain. NGF helps your dendrites connect with and receive information from other neurons, thereby helping you store and receive memories. Or as psychologist John Arden puts it: "The more input, the better the memory."[35]

Aaron P. Nelson, the Harvard Medical School doctor and author of the *Harvard Medical School Guide to Achieving an Optimal Memory,* similarly recommends getting regular exercise, noting that those who engage in vigorous exercise regularly "tend to stay mentally sharp into their seventies and eighties and beyond."[36] While you don't need to run a marathon, you should do something to get your heart beating faster or get you sweating, such as jogging, walking, or gardening, at least three times a week.

Exercise increases your brain's facility in several ways, according to a study by University of Illinois researchers, published in 2004. They found that exercise increases the capillary growth around the neurons, which enables the blood to bring more oxygen and nutrients to the brain. Also, exercise increases the density of the synapses, which are involved in transferring information from cell to cell.[37] Additionally, according to Dr. Gary Small, Director of the UCLA Center on Aging who wrote *The Memory Bible,* physical exertion increases the circulation of endorphins, hormones released in the brain after exercise, that improve both your mood and your memory. You feel a kind of mildly euphoric "endorphin boost" that gives you more energy and stimulates your brain.[38]

So what can you do to get more exercise? Some of these are suggested by Nelson:

- When you can, jog instead of walking; walk or ride a bike instead of driving.
- Walk around the neighborhood for about a half-hour at home or at work.
- Walk up the stairs instead of taking an elevator.
- Create a home exercise routine with different types of exercises, such as aerobics, weight training, and Pilates.
- Participate in an exercise class.
- Join a health club.
- Participate in a sport that involves physical exercise, such as swimming, tennis, running, or bike riding.

- Go dancing.
- Go hiking or birding or rock collecting—anything that gets you up and out and keeps you moving.

It's important to ease into doing any physical exertion, so be sure to warm up. And check with your doctor, if you haven't been physically active for awhile, to see what you can reasonably do.

A Matter of Mood and Emotions

Finally, anything you can do to have a good mood or a good attitude will help your brain power, since a negative state—such as feeling stressed, depressed, anxious, or fearful—will detract from your mental processing. Why? Because you will feel less energy or be distracted by whatever you feel upset about.

There is also a triggering effect in that a bad mood can lead you to feel apathetic and lack interest in things, so you withdraw from enriching environments, according to Karen Markowitz and Eric Jensen. Lack of enrichment causes the brain cells to deteriorate and show fewer connections via the dendrites and synapses, because you are not continuing to challenge yourself intellectually.[39] Additionally, feeling bad for an extended time can cause you to have an imbalance of neurotransmitters in the brain. Since these transmitters are involved in acquiring, consolidating, and retrieving memories, this imbalance will reduce your ability to perform these tasks.[40]

So if you are feeling bad, seek to get back into a positive mood state, and in the process you will get your brain back to the proper chemical balance for having a better memory. While some people try to do this by using alcohol or drugs, we have seen that this is not the way to go. What you can do to put yourself in a better mood is to use mental imagery and visualization, as well as engaging in some activity that makes you feel good. For example, take some time out to engage in an activity you like; talk to other people; set up a new positive goal to work toward; or create a positive enjoyable environment, such as by playing music you like and putting out flowers or candles.

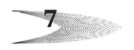

Decrease Stress and Anxiety to Remember More

Stress is common in today's workplace because of the pressures of our competitive, success-oriented age. These constant pressures to perform well, meet deadlines, and be successful can interfere with your ability to remember. Certainly a little stress can be stimulating and encourage people to do even better, such as when a speaker feels a twinge of anxiety before giving a talk and does very well, because that small amount of stress has triggered extra adrenalin, giving the speaker more energy and more motivation for performance. But when the stress level gets too high, it interferes with performance—and affects the memory required for performing. In some cases, high stress may even make performing impossible. Rather than pushing you to peak performance, the intense anxiety blocks a good performance.

By the same token, if you worry a little about meeting a deadline, that worry can stimulate you to get moving and do what needs to be done. But if you have too many worries or small worries get out of hand, it can lead to a vicious cycle in which these negative thoughts become the focus of your attention. They not only shut out the creative, productive thoughts that contribute to accomplishing the goal, but they distract you and cause you to forget.

Thus, learning to relax and getting rid of unwanted tension becomes critical for working effectively and achieving an optimal memory. The key to keeping this tension at bay is to watch for signs that you are overly tense or overstressed. Then, work on creating an appropriate balance between the slight tension needed to stimulate an effective performance, where you are sharp in remembering what you need to, and being sufficiently relaxed to feel confident and composed, so you carry out any task smoothly and efficiently.

Four Steps to Reducing Stress

There are four steps to reducing and eliminating unwanted stress and tension. Select the relaxation or stress reduction techniques that feel most comfortable for you. I have adapted the following material about relaxation techniques from my book *Mind Power: Picture Your Way to Success*.

These four steps are:

1. Calm down with a relaxation technique.
2. Understand the sources of your stress or tension.
3. Decide what to do to get rid of this source of stress or tension.
4. Chase away any worries about the problem.

Calm Down with a Relaxation Technique

You can use any number of relaxation techniques. Work with these techniques at first in a quiet place until you feel comfortable with them. Then, you can do them anywhere—even in a crowd or noisy office; you just have to concentrate harder.

Four calming approaches are as follows:

- Focus on your breath to shift your attention from the distractions and stresses of the outer world to the peaceful inner world.
- Quiet your body to quiet your mind.
- Concentrate on a soothing visual image or sound to calm both your body and mind.

- Develop a stress-reduction trigger to calm yourself when you feel pressure.

Use whichever of these four approaches suits you best, or combine them as you wish.

Focus on Your Breath

Use your breathing to calm yourself down.

Begin by paying attention to your breathing. Notice your breath going in and out, in and out. Experience the different parts of your body moving up and down, in and out, as you breathe.

With each breath, direct your breath to a different point in your body. Breathe down to your foot, to your hand, and feel your breath flowing in and out.

Now consciously breathe slowly and deeply for ten breaths. As you do, say to yourself: "I am relaxed. I am relaxed."

You should now be relaxed. To get even more so, continue using this, or use another relaxation exercise.

Quiet Your Body

Use muscle tension and a feeling of warmth to calm down.

To begin, tighten all your muscles as tight as you can. Clench your fists, your feet, your arms, your legs, your stomach muscles. Clench your teeth; squinch up your face; tense everything. Then release and relax all your muscles as much as you can. Just let everything go, and be aware of the difference. Do this three times.

Now, beginning with your feet and working your way up to your head, concentrate on each body part getting warm and relaxed. As you do, say to yourself: "My [toes, feet, legs, thighs] are now warm and relaxed." Do this sequentially for each body part.

As you do this, you may become aware of certain tensions or tightness in certain body areas. If so, you can send healing energy to that part of your body.

Continue relaxing each body part in turn. After you have relaxed your head, conclude the exercise by saying to yourself: "Now I am totally calm, totally relaxed, totally ready to experience whatever comes."

Concentrate on a Calming Image or Sound

Use images and sounds to slow yourself down.

There are innumerable calming images and sounds on which you can concentrate. Here are a few possibilities.

- Visualize yourself entering an elevator. Push one of the buttons to descend. As you pass each floor, you become more and more relaxed, more and more relaxed. When you are fully relaxed, step out of the elevator feeling calm and refreshed.
- Visualize yourself by the seashore. Notice the waves and watch them flow in and out, in and out, in and out. As they do, feel yourself becoming calmer and calmer. Then, when you feel fully calm, leave the shore.
- Chant a single syllable or sound like "om" or "ah." As you do this, experience the sound expanding in your head, erasing all other distracting images and thoughts.

Develop a Stress-Reduction Trigger

Another key to relaxing when you suddenly feel stressed is to develop a stress-reduction trigger for yourself. Then, whenever you feel sensations of stress coming on, you can catch yourself and remain calm and relaxed. To create this trigger, end your relaxation exercise with a suggestion that whenever you want to relax, you will do one of the following:

- Bring together the thumb and middle forefinger of your right hand.
- Say to yourself several times: "I am calm. I am relaxed."
- Create your own triggering device that suggests relaxation to you.

Once you have created your trigger, you can use it whenever you feel under pressure, to help yourself calm down. For instance, suppose you are nervous about an important strategy meeting with your boss. Just before the meeting is a good time to use your trigger to tell yourself you feel calm and relaxed. Or you might tell yourself you feel confident; or perhaps mentally picture the meeting going exactly as you want, so you are more likely to get the outcome you want.

While these relaxation approaches help to calm you down and relieve mild symptoms of stress, they don't deal with the underlying reasons you are feeling stressed. So for a deeper, more permanent solution, seek to understand what you are doing to make yourself tense, and learn how to get rid of this source of tension by coming up with alternative actions. You'll find your memory will improve as the things causing you to feel stress diminish.

Understand the Sources of Your Stress or Tension

To find out the reason you feel tense, get in a relaxed frame of mind and mentally ask yourself the question, "Why am I so tense right now?" Then, listen to whatever thoughts pop into your mind or notice any images that appear. These spontaneous messages will give you insights into your inner feelings and concerns.

If you have any difficulty getting a full response to your question, you can spur your inner processes in two ways:

- Imagine that you are talking to an inner guide or counselor, or that you are getting the information you seek on a computer console or movie screen.
- Write down any thoughts or images on a sheet of paper using an automatic writing process to make your thoughts flow more freely.

Decide What to Do to Get Rid of This Source of Tension

Once you have determined the reason for your stress in a particular situation, ask yourself what to do about it, drawing on your answers from your inner self. To do so, while you are still in this relaxed state, ask a question about what steps to take now, such as: "What do I need to do to stay calm?" Again, don't try to shape your answer consciously, but be receptive to what your inner mind tells you.

Then, to get more information, ask a further question: "What else must I do to stay calm?"

The key to getting the answer is to encourage your inner spontaneity to tell you what you need to know. Once again, use an inner guide, counselor, screen, or automatic writing to encourage the process, if you encounter any resistance to your question.

Chase Away Any Worries About the Problem

The final step is to chase away any worries and fears about achieving the results you want. These worries are like an internal negative dialogue we have with ourselves in which we state all the "can'ts" preventing us from doing something, or we express our fears about why what we want won't occur. But such concerns are totally unproductive and only increase the feelings of stress that interfere with your memory.

For instance, take that important strategy meeting mentioned previously: You may already feel anxious and tense, as you consider it very important to make a good impression. But worries take away your inner confidence that you can do it, as they lead you to focus on such concerns as "Maybe I can't," "Maybe I won't be good enough," and the like.

In turn, as your worries lead you to churn the situation over and over in your mind and fear that the event won't turn out successfully, they not only make you feel terrible, but they distract you from what you need to remember to make the event go well. So these negative thoughts contribute to creating the very outcome you fear. For instance, if you're worried that you won't give a good presentation, you probably won't. You'll not only lack the confidence you need, but you will likely forget what you want to say and your whole manner will convey the impression: "I don't think I'm any good." Furthermore, your worries can interfere with using the methods described here to relieve stress, as they lead you to think these techniques won't work.

In short, as you worry and feel more stress, filling your mind with negative thoughts and emotions, you will be distracted and remember less, further undermining your performance. Thus, learning to relax—or as the saying goes, "Don't worry. Be happy"—will help you remember more and allow you to do better at whatever you want to do.

Overcoming Worries and Fears

So how do you overcome any worries or fears that are making you feel stressed out and tense? You can eliminate them in four ways:

1. Come up with an alternative, so you can act to affect the situation.
2. Visualize the outcome you want, and your focus on this will help bring about the desired result.
3. Remind yourself that you will do it, in order to build your confidence.
4. Affirm that whatever happens is what should happen, so you can accept what comes and feel satisfied with it.

Depending on the situation, use any one or a combination of these techniques. Afterwards, turn your thoughts to something else, unless you have planned a specific action, so you continue to keep your attention away from your worries and fears.

Come Up with an Alternative

See yourself as the director of a movie. You are sitting in your director's chair on a film set, which is in the same location as where you are having your current problem. You also have a script in your hands, which is about this problem. The actors are waiting in the wings for their cue to start playing out this script, and one of the characters represents you.

Now, as you watch for a few moments, the characters act out the events leading up to the present situation. For example, if this is a work problem, the actors will be your boss, work associates, or employees. If you are worried about a business deal, you will see yourself in negotiations with the principal players. The characters play the scene just as you have remembered it.

As the action comes to the present time, the actor playing you goes over to the director and asks: "What does the script say I should do now?"

Listen to the reply. The director (your inner voice) may have several suggestions that you can try. Or he may tell you to wait and relax. If the director is uncertain, this tells you that you should do nothing actively now to affect the situation (although you can visualize the outcome you want or affirm your willingness to accept whatever comes).

Whatever the results, feel you can trust this inner voice, so there is no need to worry any longer. Then you can act, wait, or relax as suggested, and feel confident that the appropriate outcome will occur.

Visualize the Desired Outcome

If you already know the outcome you would like, visualize it occurring to make those results more likely. For example, if you want your co-workers to go along with your suggestions at a meeting, see yourself presenting a forceful argument and see them agreeing with what you have to say. Meanwhile, as you see this outcome, feel confident it will happen, so you can put any worries about the results out of your mind.

To reinforce your visualization, use the following telegram technique:

See yourself in a private office at work. Even if you don't currently have a private office, imagine that you do, and it is very comfortable and quiet. Now, imagine it is the present and you are thinking about the situation that has been bothering you. Suddenly, there is a knock on the door. You get up, answer it, and a messenger hands you an overnight envelope, which says on it in big red letters: "Urgent and important."

You open the envelope, read it, and feel ecstatic, because the letter informs you that everything is the way you would like it to be. For example, if you are concerned about a presentation, you are giving a good one. If you are worried about a promotion, you are getting it. If you are having problems with a co-worker, all is resolved.

Now, for the next few minutes, concentrate on seeing the desired situation before you. You have exactly what you want.

Remind Yourself You Will Do It

You can also chase away your fears about something you have to do by building up your confidence that you can do it. A simple way to do this is to remind yourself from time to time during the day that you can and will do it.

Take a few quiet minutes now and then to get calm and centered and say to yourself several times, with intense concentration:

"I can do it (fill in the image of whatever you want to do). I am doing it (fill in the image of yourself doing it)."

The key is to see yourself doing whatever you wish to do in the here and now, so your inner mind gets used to your doing it. Also, feel a sense of assurance and confidence that you are doing this activity correctly and effectively. Perhaps visualize others being pleased and complimenting you on whatever you have done (such as writing a good report, giving a good presentation, leading a successful meeting).

You'll feel better immediately. You'll be calmer, more relaxed, less worried about whatever you have to do. In addition, when it comes time to perform the activity, you'll do it better, because you feel more confident and you have already rehearsed it in your mind.

Affirm Your Acceptance

Sometimes, no matter how much you try to actively or mentally influence events, circumstances may not turn out as you hoped. You don't get a desired transfer or promotion; you suddenly find an expected client doesn't come through. Yet, often, in the long run, things will turn out for the best, if you are only patient.

Thus, one important key to overcoming worries is to realize that often things may seem to go wrong, but you can turn them around or use what goes wrong as a learning experience to create something even better. Still another way to think of initially undesirable events is to realize that often your wants and needs differ, and when they do, you usually get what you need. For example, a person longs for a new job title with additional responsibilities and a new office. But, in fact, the person hasn't had sufficient experience to handle the job, and would find herself over her head and perhaps fired if she were promoted right away.

Thus, it is important to develop a feeling of acceptance about whatever happens, as well as trying to do your best to achieve your goals. In other words, if you truly feel you have done everything possible to attain a goal but don't reach it, accept this outcome. The important thing is you have done your all, and now it's time to be receptive and patient until the next opportunity presents itself.

The value of this approach is that you are aligning yourself with the flow of events, rather than fighting against the current. Further, you are basing your actions on the premise that nothing in the universe happens by coincidence, but rather the universe seems to respond to our needs by providing exactly what we require. Thus, what happens is what should happen.

In turn, if you use this premise to guide your life, you will find everything much easier for you. You'll still try as hard as you can to attain your goals. Yet you'll also feel a sense of satisfaction and completion regardless of what happens, knowing that somehow you can profit from the experience and consider it to be for the best in the long run.

The following visualization will help you develop this power of acceptance.

> *See yourself seated in a park near where you work. The sun is shining brightly, and it is very quiet and peaceful. You are enjoying a lunch break, and you feel very calm, relaxed, and receptive to whatever comes.*
>
> *Now, from the distance, some people arrive carrying small, wrapped packages tied with ribbons. They come over to you and hand you the packages as a gift.*
>
> *As you open each package you find a different present inside. It may be some money, an object, a certificate providing some service to you. Some gifts you want, others you need, others are unexpected. But as you open each gift, you receive it with the same spirit of equal acceptance, and you say simply to the person who gave it to you: "Thank you, I accept."*
>
> *You continue receiving these gifts, until all of the gift bearers have finished giving them to you and leave.*
>
> *Remind yourself that these gifts represent the experiences and challenges you encounter in life. And just like you have received and accepted each gift, you must receive and accept each experience that comes like a gift. You must participate to the best of your ability, and use the experi-*

ence to learn from and grow. But whatever it is, you must learn to accept it.

For this is the secret of staying calm and relaxed, overcoming stress, and getting rid of worries. You must learn to receive and accept, as well as try to achieve and grow.

Stress and Memory

When you are stressed out, you may not even realize all of the ways in which your mind and body are affected. However, you can easily recognize this connection between tension and memory, if you stop and think about a time when your memory failed because you were overly anxious. For example, your boss suddenly asks you for a key fact or number during a big, highly anticipated meeting; you freeze up and can't remember it—even though you knew it well the night before. But if a co-worker asks you the same question while passing in the hall, you easily recall the information and immediately provide the right answer.

Reducing stress and tension through the techniques discussed here will help you improve your memory dramatically. Just by maintaining a calm, focused attitude toward whatever you are doing, you will be able eliminate or reduce the negative effects of intense anxiety so you can perform at your best.

8

Increase Your Energy to Boost Your Memory Power

Just as your overall health contributes to your ability to remember, so does your level of energy. If you are tired, sleepy, groggy, or otherwise feeling lethargic and low in energy, you are just not going to be able to remember well.

Some classic examples of when your flagging energy interferes with memory are when you are cramming to remember something at a late-night review session before a critical meeting or when you are studying for an exam. Your feelings of fatigue will simply get in the way of your remembering. They will reduce your ability at all levels of the memory process—from focusing your attention to encoding information in your brain to retrieving the information later. No matter what you are doing, if you are tired and feeling low in energy, you won't perform as well—and trying to remember something is no different.

But what if you still feel tired at times, despite doing what you can to maintain a high level of health, including eating and sleeping well? Then, there are assorted techniques you can use to increase your energy on the spot, and thereby boost your memory power. These techniques aren't a cure-all for other problems causing you to feel low in energy. If you continue to feel an energy low for an extended time, you should take other measures, among them seeing a doctor. But on an occasional or as-needed basis, you can use these techniques to give yourself a dramatic energy surge, which is what you need for better memory power.

For example, John, a freelance writer and designer, uses these energy techniques when he has an unusually large number of clients or deadlines, so he can handle all of the extra work in order to offset the slow periods in an often unpredictable business. They help him to revive his flagging spirits and recharge himself to get through the occasional late-night assignments that he has to turn in the next day. Instead of using stimulants or energy boosters, he uses the abilities of his mind to renew himself so that he can keep going and get everything done.

Similarly, Maggie, a secretary in a large office, finds that using mental imagery techniques, rather than filling up on coffee or pastries to give her an energy charge, is a healthier way to get a boost, especially after a late-night date or party leaves her feeling unmotivated the next day at work.

Likewise, when you need a quick energy fix to overcome feelings of fatigue and motivate yourself to do something, you can use these energy-boosting techniques. And then your increased energy will turn into greater memory power, too. These techniques are ideal in the following types of situations:

- You feel draggy or sleepy during the day.
- You have to start a big project and feel overwhelmed by all you have to do, so you resist getting started.
- You don't feel motivated to work on a project, although you know you have to do it.
- You have to come up with some ideas for a project and feel your creative energy is blocked.
- You have to be alert and enthusiastic for some activity, such as making a sales call, giving a speech, or leading a meeting.
- You need something to get you going in the morning and keep you going at night.

These energy booster techniques work, in the situations above or whenever you need a quick charge, because you are using your imagination and thoughts to create the energy you need. As a result, you don't need to use anything artificial like pep pills, which can upset your body chemistry and have unpleasant side effects. Instead, you are drawing the energy you need from inside you, from the energy of the earth and air around you, or from a combination of these sources—whatever concept feels best for you.

Using Different Energy-Raising Approaches

These energy-raising techniques are based on directing your attention and imagination to some image or experience that leaves you feeling more energized.

One way is to use self-talk, sometimes accompanied by a short physical exercise, to think energy-raising thoughts. Another approach is to imagine that you have columns of energy flowing into and through you. Then, too, you can imagine yourself participating in some enjoyable energetic activity.

Certainly, at times, you can use actual physical exercise to up your energy, such as going for a short hike or taking a quick swim to recharge yourself—as long as you don't exert yourself too much, so you feel even more tired after your exercise. Or perhaps going for a short massage or taking a midday nap can renew your energy. But sometimes you don't have the luxury of getting away to increase your energy, such as when you need that energy boost just before a meeting or before you have to plunge into a difficult task on the computer. That's when using a visualization technique works very well. You can't get up and out—but you certainly can perk yourself up.

The following techniques will rouse you to do whatever you have to do.

- *Create your own energy and enthusiasm.* This technique is particularly good for a situation in which you need a quick rush of energy to wake up, keep going, or feel more enthusiastic and motivated.

- *Draw on the energies of the universe.* This technique is ideal if you have to generate the energy or creative spark to work on a big project.
- *Imagine yourself doing something exciting.* This last technique works especially well if you are feeling generally lethargic or your mood is low; it not only increases your energy, but improves your mood.

Creating Your Own Energy and Enthusiasm (Time: about 1 minute)

This is a technique in which you combine self-talk with a short physical burst of activity to feel a quick renewal.

> *Stand with your feet slightly apart and make a fist with one hand. Then, quickly raise your hand to your head and lower it several times. Each time you bring it down, shout out something like: "I am awake," "I feel energetic," "I am enthusiastic and excited," or "I am raring to get up and go." Do this five to ten times.*
>
> *As you do this, feel a rush of energy and enthusiasm surge through you, and soon you'll be awake and alert and ready to tackle any project.*

If other people are around so you can't actively participate in this exercise, imagine yourself doing it in your mind's eye. It's more stimulating to use your whole body, but using your power of mental imagery alone will help wake you up or motivate you to act.

Drawing on the Energies of the Universe (Time: 2–3 minutes)

In this technique, you imagine the energies of the earth and the cosmos coursing through you to give you the energy you need to do something you want to do. The reason for drawing on these two different energies is that you can imagine the energy of the earth as more solid and grounding and the energy of the air or cosmos as more light and expansive. Then, you combine a visualization of these two energies with your own energy to create a single, blended pulse of energy. You can use the interplay of these two different types of energy to draw on the energy you feel you need most.

You can think of the energy-raising process in hard science

terms, based on the physics principle that everything in the universe is made up of molecules of energy. As a result, when these energy molecules come together to form material objects, this includes you, and your thoughts are waves of energy, too. The ability of thought to move matter is shown by some of recent experiments in which subjects have been able to maneuver a cursor on a computer just by thinking where they want that cursor to go. At the lower theta, delta, and alpha frequencies of our brain waves, which are associated with sleep and meditation, our thoughts move more slowly, while at the beta frequency associated with everyday thinking, we are more active and alert. In turn, the frequencies of our thoughts can influence the frequencies of our bodies.

Thus, when you use your mind powers to concentrate on raising your energy level, you are actually stimulating the molecules of energy in your body to move more quickly, so you not only feel more energetic but become more energetic. By the same token, when you focus on drawing in energy from the universe, the imagery of this energy serves to activate your body.

So now get ready to use this energy of the universe to increase your own energy levels.

Begin by sitting with your spine straight, your feet on the floor, your hands up to receive the energy, and your eyes closed.

Now see the energy of the earth coming up through the ground and surging into your body. Feel it rising through your feet, through your legs, to the base of your spine, and expanding out through your torso, into your arms and head. Feel its strength in your arms and head. Feel its strength and its power.

Meanwhile, as the earth energy surges through you, see the energy of the universe coming in through the top of your head, into your spine, into your arms, and spiraling down through your torso. Notice that this energy feels light, airy, expansive.

Then, focus on the two energies meeting at the base of your spine, and see them join and spiral around together—moving up and down your spine and filling you with energy. You can balance the two energies, if you wish, by drawing on extra energy from the earth (heavy) or from the universe (light) as needed.

Keep running this energy up and down your spine until you feel filled with energy.

Now, if you have a project or task you want to do, direct this energy toward doing this project. If you haven't felt motivated to do it, notice that you feel motivated and excited to begin work on this project now. If you have been resisting doing something because there is so much to do, be aware that you now have the energy and enthusiasm to tackle the project, and you feel confident you can do it. If you have felt your creativity blocked, experience your creative juices flowing now, and know that you are able to perform this task.

As you direct this energy, see it flowing out of you as needed so you can do this project. For example, if you want to write or type something, visualize the energy surging out through your hands. If you plan to lift some heavy objects, visualize the energy coming out through your feet, body, and hands. Whatever you need to do, see the energy coursing through you as needed, so you can do whatever you want to do.

After you finish this exercise, plunge immediately into your project. You'll find you suddenly have lots of energy and enthusiasm.

Imagining Yourself Doing Something Exciting (Time: 5–10 minutes)

In this technique, you raise your energy by imagining you are doing something fun and exciting. It could be something you already do, say if you go hiking or sailing. Or you might imagine yourself engaging in some sport or other physical activity that you have never tried before but that appeals to you.

In either case, project yourself into the experience as intensely as possible. For example, if you are skiing, see yourself up in the mountains and look around you and savor the view. Then, as you whiz down, reassuring yourself that you will be completely safe, see the snow, trees, and other people you pass on the slope. Feel the cool wind in your face. Experience the vibration of the ground under your feet. And so on. In short, whatever you do, put yourself into the scene like an actor in a film and then truly experience everything as if you are in the scene; don't just watch.

Some examples of things to experience might be dancing, ice

skating, roller skating, going on a carnival ride, parachuting or hang-gliding, surfing, or mountain climbing—whatever turns you on.

The Power of These Techniques

Any of these techniques, individually or in combination, can be really powerful. I have found them invaluable for raising energy in my own work. For example, when I first started writing—initially for clients before I began writing my own books—I used the energies of the universe technique to start my day, so I felt ready and motivated to write. I knew I had to meet certain deadlines and wanted to be sure to meet them.

Thus, each morning, before going to write, I began by sitting in my living room and visualizing the energy pouring into me and swirling around through me. Then I pictured it pouring out of me into the writing assignment I had for that day. As a result, I went to the typewriter—yes, we used typewriters in those days!—feeling charged up, confident I could do whatever was required, and enthusiastic and motivated to get to work right away. After a few weeks I had conditioned myself to begin working every time I went to the typewriter, so I no longer needed to continue doing the exercises. But initially, this technique proved invaluable in getting me energized and self-motivated to work on a regular writing schedule and it enabled me to complete my assignments successfully.

Then, I began to apply the technique in other situations, such as giving a class or seminar, to feel upbeat and inspired; in those kinds of cases, I imagine the energy pouring through me and coming out through my voice. I found these techniques worked well as a quick pick-me-up during the day and they helped me when I was doing sales for a while to help me feel more energetic and enthusiastic when I went to the phone, since in sales you face a lot of no's before getting a yes.

Similarly, you might apply and adapt these techniques to suit your own situation. So take some time now to think about the times when you need more energy. When might you use these techniques? And where might you go to apply them? You can use the chart shown here to write down when and where you might apply these techniques. Then, use the chart as a reminder to use the techniques under those circumstances. Eventually, you won't have to think about using a particular technique to raise your energy—you will just find yourself tapping into a well of energy within yourself, like having a flow of lava on call when you push a button; then watch it erupt. But initially, you have to be mindful and pay attention, just like learning any new skill, until it becomes automatic—the same way the process of remembering anything works.

So now, mindfully start thinking about using these techniques; then let yourself go so you brainstorm possibilities. Just write down whatever comes to you; later you can decide where to apply these techniques when you are in that situation or setting.

TIMES WHEN I NEED MORE ENERGY		
Energy Technique	When I Might Use This Technique	Where I Might Use This Technique

A final caution. These techniques aren't designed to replace the sleep you need. If you keep drifting off while doing something and find you frequently or continually feel tired, you obviously need more sleep, or perhaps need to eat more to raise your blood sugar level. But on a short-term basis, any of these techniques is ideal for a quick energy fix.

Energy and Memory

High energy levels and good memory go hand in hand. Stories abound of students who stay up all night cramming for a test and arrive in the exam room with little or no energy. All or most of the information they studied the night before is gone; try as they may, they can't retrieve it. As a result, they wind up with a poor or failing grade. On the other hand, students with the same level of knowledge who show up for the exam well rested with lots of energy do much better—despite avoiding the all-night study sessions.

You can apply the same principle to giving an important presentation at work. You are far better off exercising and getting to bed early than trying to absorb a massive amount of data the night before. Then you can use whichever energy-boosting techniques work best for you in the morning. You will be much sharper during your presentation and better able to answer questions and provide facts and figures on the spot, rather than fumbling through your talk and forgetting key bits of information.

All of the techniques described here will help you to boost your energy level when it flags. As you master these techniques, you'll find that increasing your energy will help you maintain a good memory and contribute to further improve your memory as you work on other memory improvement techniques.

9

It's All About Me!

The self-referent effect is an important one for making memories. Whether it draws your attention or helps you encode a memory, the more you can tie something you want to remember to yourself, the better you will remember it. You might call this the "looking after number one principle" or the "numero uno effect." We call it the "all about me principle"—and it really works.

The All About Me Principle

The all about me principle is the principle used in any selling—show the customer the benefit so he or she will buy, because people want to know, "What's in it for me?" Well, that's how it works with your memory, too. If something seems important to you personally, you will be more likely to remember it—and you'll remember it more vividly and in greater detail.

According to the self-referent effect, "You will remember more information if you try to relate that information to yourself."[1] A reason for this is that the connection to yourself means whatever you are doing or trying to remember is more meaningful for you. As a result, when you encode the experience or item into memory, you are doing more of what psychologists call "deep processing," where you think about other associations, images, and past experiences related to the stimulus, which all contribute to making this experience or item meaningful. For example, psychologists repeatedly have found that people are more likely to recall something that applies to themselves than something that doesn't.[2]

This me-me-me effect is so powerful for a number of reasons. You find what you want to remember is more meaningful to you if it's about you. You are answering the question: "Why the heck should I be interested in this?" You are also more likely to think about it—or "rehearse" it, as the psychologists call this process. Moreover, psychologists have found that when you engage in deep processing, you activate certain regions of the brain, most notably the left and right prefrontal cortex, associated with recall.[3]

You have probably experienced this phenomenon repeatedly in your own life. For example:

• You remember to pick up tickets for a concert you really want to go to—and you remember the names of the main performers.

• You remember the name and location of a store that has a new, hip product you really want to buy.

• You remember the prices of items you are really interested in buying, so if the clerk makes a mistake, you point this out.

• You remember to call someone for a reference for that really important job you are interviewing for.

Take a few minutes to think about all the things you have remembered recently because they were important to you. In many cases, you may not have realized you paid extra attention or absorbed this information while you went about the day on automatic. But when you needed the information, you just called it up, and it was there.

You can write down these important things you have remembered on the chart below. As you write them down, think about how much easier it was to remember them than something else that wasn't important to you. Then, just for comparison, write down some things you didn't remember that weren't particularly important to you. (Since you don't remember, just write down the category of what you tried to think of that you couldn't remember—such as "name of a book," "title of film," or "political figure in the news.")

REMEMBERING WHAT'S IMPORTANT TO ME	
What I Have Remembered Recently That's Important to Me	**What I Have Forgotten Recently That's Not Important to Me**

After you write down items on your list, compare them. Notice the difference in the way your memory came to your aid when something was very important to you, but often slipped away when you weren't particularly interested—even when you were exposed to that experience or idea and others around you were talking about it.

So to remember more, be self-centered! Think about how whatever you are trying to learn or remember relates to you. When you do, not only will you be more likely to remember, but you may gain additional benefits for yourself, such as finding ways in which something or someone can be a valuable asset to you, increase your profits, expand your network, and so on.

Applying the All About Me Principle

Following are some ways to put the all about me principle into practice in different situations. As you do, consider how you might combine this approach with other techniques you use to remember, such as using image associations, chunking large amounts of information together into smaller groups, and rehearsing through repetition.

- *You have met someone at an event.* Think about how that person could help you—or how you might help that person, which in turn could help you later with more referrals and business. You might also think about any associations you have with that contact, such as belonging to the same club, knowing someone in common, dressing in a similar way, traveling to the same place, liking the same vacation spot, working for the same company or in the same industry, and so on. Whatever you do to help you bond with that person and assess how you might do business or network together in the future will build additional memory traces that will help you recall who that person is later.

- *You have learned some information in a course.* Think about how whatever you are learning might apply in your own life. For instance, if you learn about economic trends, imagine how those will affect your own buying power as a consumer. If you learn about people living in another society with different customs and beliefs, think about what customs and beliefs you share in common or how any differences might be helpful to you. If you learn about the features of a new tech product, consider how you would use that product yourself and how that might affect your life.

- *You have heard someone introduce some new programs for your company at a meeting.* Think about how those programs might affect you and your department in the company.

So now, take it away, and come up with some other ways in which you might apply these types of information and experiences to yourself. To further remember these applications, don't just think them. Write them down.

OTHER WAYS I CAN APPLY THE ALL ABOUT ME PRINCIPLE	
Type of Situation	How I Can Apply It to Me

Then, with this awareness of the different circumstances in which you might apply the all about me principle, apply it in your everyday life. Afterwards, reflect on the experience and notice how it has been working for you. How has the technique increased your memory for the situations where you have applied it? And what other gains have you experienced, such as improved relationships, increased business, and greater productivity? You might include your observations in your memory journal.

10

Remembering More by
Remembering Less

It may seem like a paradox, but one way to remember more is to remember less. In other words, you can set up systems to help you remember a lot of less important details, so that you can better focus on what's more important to you. Moreover, you can use these systems to help remind you of things that are important to remember now.

You may be familiar with at least some of these systems, such as the age-old advice to put a string around your finger to remind you to do something (though this doesn't work very well if you see the string and don't remember what it's for). Other commonly used systems include creating files for storing important information in one place; setting up tickler files, which provide a reminder to do something on a particular day or date; keeping daily and weekly calendars; placing Post-its on a bulletin board or the refrigerator; or creating a shopping list or to-do list.

The reason for creating these systems is that we are so bombarded with information, you can't remember everything—and don't even want to. These systems enable you to move information off your desk into a folder, up on a bulletin board, or onto a list, so you reduce the litter. Then, as needed, you can locate that information. You don't need to keep it in the forefront of your memory now, and therefore you can clear out some space for what is more important.

Following are a variety of reminder and retrieval systems you can set up. Use the ones that are most suitable for you.

Creating a Passwords File

Today, everyone has passwords for everything—from e-mail to bank accounts to online subscriptions to payment accounts. And many services advise you to change your password from time to time, so you are better protected.

Some people use the same or a limited number of passwords for everything, and if they change them, they apply these changes to everything with the same password. But this approach doesn't always work, since some companies have different formats for passwords and some may assign you a password when you sign up. Then there are the really long numbers for registration codes that are all but impossible to remember.

A good way to deal with all these passwords is to keep a file handy where you put your passwords—and just in case, keep a copy of this file in another safe place. While you may remember some of the commonly used passwords you use everyday, the file is an ideal place to store the passwords you rarely use—or the really long ones that can fry your brain if you struggle to encode them.

When you create such a file, you might print out a page for each company and password you need to remember; then for easy retrieval, store them by type of company (i.e., banks, writers, Websites) and alphabetically. Or alternatively, you can create a Word or Excel document with this list, though the extra time to do this may not be necessary.

Later, when you are asked for a password and don't remember it, just pull out your file.

Creating a File for Lock Combinations

If you have combinations for locks or lockboxes, write these down, too. However, for security purposes, it might be better to keep these filed separately from your passwords. When you use these combinations each day, you may be able to readily remember them. But after a while, if you don't use them, the combination will usually fade away.

As with passwords, it's a good idea to keep this information in two places—a file where you put all your combinations and a copy in another safe place. Also, be sure to carefully note which combination goes to what, particularly when you have several locks or lockboxes with different combinations. For example, you might distinguish them by the place where you have put that particular lock or box, such as Rear Door Lock: R3, L20, R7; Side Door Lock: L4, R8, L23.

Using a Keyword Reminder

Aside from creating a password or combination file to remind you what these are, you might also create a keyword to remind you what password or combination you have used. Even Website services that require a password to enter use this principle. For instance, if you use your dog's name with a set of numbers for one password, your keyword might be "Dog." If you use your mother's last name and other numbers for another password, your keyword might be "Mom." Such a reminder might be ideal when you are in a situation where you aren't able to refer to your file or don't want to, such as when you are working in a public place and don't want to take the chance that someone might take this extremely confidential file. This approach is particularly ideal if you have a single password or combination that you use for one type of activity and another password or combination for another activity. This keyword can then tell you which password or combination you used.

Creating a Tickler File

A good way to remember particular events or activities that you have to do at a certain time is to create a tickler file—either a physical one or one set up on your computer, such as in Microsoft Outlook or another calendar program. The purpose of such a file is to organize a calendar of the tasks you have to do or the events you plan to attend on a particular date, so you will do those tasks or participate in that activity. If this file is on your computer or laptop, keep a back-up copy someplace, so if your computer crashes, you will have another copy. Or keep a hard-copy version as your back-up.

In some cases, it will work well to have a master calendar, where you enter everything for the day and time when you expect to do it. But sometimes it is helpful to organize similar activities together, such as having a tickler file for your appointments and activities at work during the day, and another for the activities in your personal life. (Just be sure that you don't have an overlap of hours if you keep separate files, or you may find you are scheduling more than one activity for the same time.)

For example, Jim, a private investigator I know, used the calendar approach when he created a file system for his cases, placing them according to the date when he had to take some action on the case. In addition, he separates these into different types of cases, so he can perform similar actions on a set of cases. Then, after he performs a particular action, he indicates what he did according to a cover sheet with rows for each date and action. Next, he moves that file ahead to a folder with the date in the future when he next has to take some action on the case. Lawyers, counselors, and others dealing with clients use a similar type of system to remind them when it's time to act on a case.

Still another approach is to use an undated filing system but group files by the particular activity to be performed. For instance, that's what I do for one of the e-mail connection businesses I've set up—PublishersAndAgents.Net, which links writers with publishers. I identified a series of tasks that have to be done in a set sequence, from getting the initial order to finalizing the query letter, sending it out, and getting a testimonial about the great service from the client. So I have a large folder for each step in the process and I keep these folders in the order in which I perform each step. Then, each day, I go through the files, take the appropriate action, make a copy of the action I have taken, staple that to the top of the file for each client, and move the whole file into the next step in the sequence. Since I put the latest action on the top of the client's file and staple everything together, I don't need a separate checklist to keep track of the step where each client is in the process. It's all readily apparent by just looking at the last action taken for that client.

I file all of each client's correspondence, which is assigned an order number and is stapled together with most recent communication on top, in the folder for that step. (For example, I have a folder for writing the letter, another for reviewing and editing a client's letter, and another for having the letter ready to go and awaiting the client's final approval.) Then, I pick out the material to be worked on from that folder and after it's done, the client's material goes in the next folder in the sequence, with the latest material stapled on top. Finally, when the order has been completed, it goes into a file of completed orders. Once a client writes in to say Great Job!, the material goes into the file to request permission to use their testimonials and once I have their permission, I add their testimonial to the Website. I use this system to keep track of orders, since I know I could easily forget where I am in the process, if I didn't have this step-by-step system telling me what I need to do for each client. The filing system provides a kind of flow chart of the series of tasks to be done, while the order numbers and clipped-together correspondence for each client indicates exactly what should be done next.

If you set up the system on your computer, you can set it to alert you within a certain number of days of the task, as well as establish a date for when you'd *like to* complete the task and when you *have to* complete it.

Using a Daily Calendar

Keeping a daily calendar is another way to stay on top of things. You may prefer to keep the daily calendar in a book—usually in a loose-leaf format so you can select a few months of events to take along with you. Other formats include pages held together on a pad with a large ring or an online calendar, such as the one offered by Microsoft Outlook. If you do go the online route, it's good to print out a copy of the calendar whenever you add something to the calendar or at least once a day if you make multiple entries in a single day just in case you have a computer crash or have trouble accessing your computer during the day. You might also include backing up your calendar with your regular computer back-up, which you should do every day or so for everything on your computer.

It's best to get a calendar with an hour-by-hour format for the workday listed on each page, along with a facing page where you can write down additional notes about each task (such as a contact number to call, an address of where to go, or items you need to purchase for that task). Then, take that calendar or the pages from it that you need with you, so you can readily refer to it.

It is also helpful to assign a particular place where you keep this when it isn't with you, so you can more easily find it to refer to it or add entries.

Putting Things in Their Place

So you don't have to remember where you put something, establish a place where you always put it—or one or two alternate spots if you can't use just one spot (such as when you have a date book you might look at either upstairs or downstairs). This way, if you remind yourself to always put that item in the proper place, you will never have to search around for it.

Many people use this approach to help them find their keys. Some people use a hook on a wall where they always hang their keys; another good place is in a small bowl by your front door, which is the approach I use.

Having a designated place for things is a good technique for anything that might be mobile, such as a wireless phone or iPod. Otherwise, you might frantically start looking for it the next time you go to use it. But if you develop the habit of consciously putting the item in its designated place, it will be there when you next want it.

Placing Reminders Along the Way

Another technique to remind yourself to do something is to use a physical reminder and put it somewhere you usually pass in order to trigger your memory.

For example, say you have to return a book to the library; put the book in full view on a shelf or cabinet you pass on the way to your car, so you will pick up the book as you go out the door. If you have to do some task in the house, like take out the garbage at night for an early morning pick-up, post a note or sign on the door to the garage where you keep the trash cans telling you to take out the garbage—or create a sign with a garbage can that says something like: "Take Me Out Tuesday Night."

Putting Out What You Need the Night Before

One of the worst times to try to remember what you need for the day is just before you have to leave and are in a rush. You can much better remember if you prepare what you need when you are more relaxed and less under pressure.

Thus, rather than trying to fight the clock and feeling stressed as you throw together what you want, locate what you expect to take with you the previous evening and put it out where you just have to pick it up as you leave. Then, to be sure you have taken everything you want, review what you have picked up to make sure you do have everything—and usually you will if you've used checklists or other memory aids. In short, do a quick double check to give you that feeling of reassurance that you do have everything. If not, get what you need.

Creating a To-Do List or Checklist

If you have more than two or three tasks to do, create a list or checklist of things to do—and if you have a series of tasks for different projects, create a separate list for each project.

If the items are all to be completed at the same time, a single-column list is fine. Additionally, if the items need to be completed over a period of time, prioritize your list, so you list first the tasks to be done first or clearly indicate next to each item their order of priority (say with a letter from A to E or a number from 1 to 5; you might prefer colored dots, such as blue for highest priority, red for next highest priority, and so on).

Should there be due dates or expected dates of completion, add a column so you can record them. Finally, show that you have completed the item with a checkmark or write in a date of completion. In the event that other people are going to participate in this task with you or do it for you, add in a column for that information, too, along with any specific details you need to check with them before the task to make sure they are going to be doing what you expect them to do. This way you have your own reminder to remind them!

Keeping Track of Cards You Collect

Have you ever collected cards at a social or business mixer, and when you look at them later that night or a few days later, you don't remember who someone was or why you picked up their card? It's a common experience, because at mixers you can meet more people if you quickly collect a card, give someone your own, and then move on.

However, once you and the cards are in a different context, you don't have the help of context cues to remind you who that person was and why you wanted to contact him or her again. So it's important to either put a note on the card as a reminder (be sure to have a pen with you so you can do this), or set up a system to place cards in the appropriate category for follow-up.

If you use a note, you can place this on the card as you talk or add your note immediately after your conversation, while the information is fresh in your mind and you don't have some retroactive interference from the next person you meet and exchange cards with. Include in your note the date you got the card, what the person does if not clear from the card, and what you should do to follow up and when. For example, a note might be something like: "7/26/06 Architect, Interested in health line." Or if you have developed a code system, you can shorten this entry (i.e., 7/26, arch, health). By keeping your note short, it will take just seconds to add to the card, so there will be minimal interference with your note taking—and you'll have the information you need at your fingertips for follow-up later.

Alternatively, obtain or create some kind of small filing folder you can carry with you for cards. For example, you might use a mini-card holder with sections or pockets for different categories of information; then pop the card you have just collected into the appropriate category. Later, pull the cards out of that section or pocket as you follow up—or add the note you might have used at the mixer at your leisure.

Using a Reminder Service

Another way to set up a reminder system is to let someone else do it for you. In fact, this has become a popular way of remembering all sorts of things, as reflected by the fact that there are over 5 million listings if you put "reminder services" into Google. These services range from Web-based services that will send you an e-mail reminder to software you install on your computer that will trigger the reminder to a local reminder phone call service.

For example, one service, Memo to Me (www.memotome.com), which calls itself the Internet's #1 reminder service, sends reminders both at home and at work. Personal reminders might be used to remind yourself about your anniversary, Grandma's birthday, an upcoming soccer game, or just to take out the trash. Work reminders might be to remind you about a meeting with a client, a weekly status meeting with reminders sent to your co-workers, a reminder to salespeople about their monthly sales projections, and reminders about deadlines. If you're away from your computer, you can set up reminders to go to your pager or mobile phone. You can even use the service to check your e-mail for new messages for you and send the messages to your pager or mobile phone, so you don't have to remember to check yourself.

Arranging for Reminders from Other People

A less high-tech version of having a service contact you with reminders is to arrange for friends, family, or co-workers to remind you of something. Certainly, you don't want to overwhelm them with a huge number of things to remember for you. But from time to time, especially for special circumstances, you might have someone you trust become your memory assistant. For example, if you are going to be out of town, you might arrange for an assistant, referral service, or a close friend or family member to call you with a reminder of things you need to do from afar. If so, give the person your daily checklist to use to give you reminders.

Setting Up an Alarm

If there's something you have to do at a certain time of the day, you can set an alarm to go off to remind you, though the type of alarm will vary depending on where you are. For instance, if you are at home, you can use an alarm clock in your bedroom or office. If you are traveling, you can use a travel alarm. Other possibilities include watches, cell phones, and Palm Pilots, which can be programmed to beep or ring or vibrate at whatever times you specify. Even a computer software program, such as Microsoft Outlook, can be programmed to send you a signal when it's the day and time to do something.

Then, once you are alerted that it's time to do something, use any other reminder tips to help you complete the task.

Putting Up a Reminder Bulletin Board

A reminder bulletin board is a good way to remind yourself about high-priority items both in the office and at home. One type of bulletin board comes with a corkboard, so you can use pins to post up your notes. Other possibilities include plain wood or cardboard boards where you use Post-it notes as reminders or use an erasable white board to write down the reminders for the day. Once the tasks are done, you can remove the notes or erase them and post or write in the next reminders.

When you use such a board, you can make items stand out or code them by the type of task using colored Post-its or pens. Or even use decorative notes and cartoons to make the board look more festive—as long as you can still clearly see the reminders. And be sure to refer to the reminder board each day or even every few hours to remind you what to do that day or in the next few hours.

Carrying a Notebook or Notepad with You

What if you get inspired about some kind of creative project or task to do? You could easily forget if you just make a mental note of your thoughts. Or you may find that it is inconvenient to try to encode the idea into long-term memory, since you want to think about something else at the time. An example might be if you get an idea while you are driving on the freeway, and need to think about where you are going and where to turn off.

One answer is to have a small notebook or notepad with you, so you can jot down your idea. Or use a tape recorder and just say your thoughts aloud. If you are driving, one possibility for recording your idea is to pull to the side of the road for a moment and write down your ideas in a small notebook. Or if you have a recorder with an omnidirectional mike, you can speak your thoughts or a few reminder keywords into it, as long as you can do this safely, while you drive. Suppose you are doing some errands, shopping, or taking a hike. You can stop wherever you are and pull your notebook or notepad out of your briefcase, pocketbook, backpack, or other carryall and write a few notes. Or find someplace quiet where you can do this, like a chair or restroom in a department store. Later, you can look at your notes and expand upon them if you wish, using this reminder to help you think more carefully about this idea.

Doing Something in Advance So You Don't Have to Remember to Do It Later

Preplanning can sometimes be the way to go so you don't have to think about doing something while you are doing something else. That's exactly what a woman who is a professional organizer did at a 7:00 A.M. breakfast meeting I attended. The parking meters operated from 8:00 A.M. to 6:00 P.M. on weekdays at the meters outside the meeting place. Most of the people meeting planned to go outside to pay for one hour just before 8:00 A.M. But the organizer paid for two and a half hours as she went in the door at 6:45—a cost of about $2 more. Why? Because, she told me, then she wouldn't have to think about remembering to pay during the meeting. This way, she could better concentrate on the meeting.

Similarly, if you have a task to do that may disrupt what you are going to be doing later, if it's feasible, take care of that task in advance so you don't have to remind yourself to do it. It's one less thing to think about remembering to do if you've already done it.

Creating an Appointments Scheduler and Results Form

Besides using a regular calendar, for special occasions create an Appointment Scheduler for each day, along with an Appointment Results (or Presentation) Form in which you can record what happened at each appointment. For example, I created a loose-leaf binder to do this when I set up appointments to meet with company owners and R&D directors at a Toy Fair and Games Manufacturing Show. I set the Appointment Scheduler up with columns for the time, company, contact, location of my meeting, and any comments, and my Appointment Results Form included the date presented, complete company information, the name of the people I met with, what I presented, and the results.

My Appointment Scheduler (though set up in a landscape format) looked like this:

APPOINTMENTS SCHEDULED DATE: _____				
Time	Company	Contact	Location	Comments
8:00				
8:30				
9:00				

And so on . . .

My Appointment Results Form looked like this:

APPOINTMENT RESULTS			
Company:		Date:	
Address:		Reviewed by:	
City, State, Zip:			
Phone:			
Fax:		E-Mail:	
Product Type	Name of Item Presented	Results	

And so on . . . Plus I included a Results Code from 1 to 5, indicating different types of requested actions.

Use your own categories and codings when you create your own forms.

Creating a Follow-Up Matrix

Another helpful reminder system is a Follow-Up Matrix, which indicates what to do to follow up on your meetings. The Matrix should include the name of the company, your contact there, the interests of the company or what type of action they want you to take, what you did and the date you did it, the results of your action, and e-mail or phone contact information for easy follow-up. For more detail, you can refer back to your Appointment Results or Presentation Form.

For example, my Follow-Up Matrix for the presentations I made using information from the above forms looked like this (though I set it up in a landscape format):

RESULTS OF MEETINGS WITH COMPANIES AT TOY FAIR				
Company	Contact	Interests	Action Taken and Results	E-Mail/ Phone

And so on . . .

Using Post-its or Cards with Reminders

Still another reminder system is using Post-its or index cards on which you write down the task or activity you are planning to do; then insert the Post-it or card into a folder by the day when you plan to act on it. Consider this a kind of tickler file using Post-its or cards. You might also use color-coded Post-Its or cards to indicate different types of tasks, and perhaps add a colored dot or a number on each

Post-It card to indicate the priority of what activity to do when. This priority could take into consideration both the importance and the deadline for completing the task. Then use this priority coding to indicate those tasks that are more important or must be completed sooner.

Creating Your Own System

Consider the above reminder systems as a repertoire of approaches you can use to create reminders and place information in these systems, so you don't have to remember the details yourself. Or create your own personalized reminder system for containing your information.

Reviewing Your Reminders

Once you set up a reminder system, it is critical to review this set-up from time to time, because otherwise you will be likely to forget what you are seeking to remind yourself about. It's not that you have an arcane coding system, but if you don't review it from time to time, you may forget what different codes refer to, such as when you are using different letters of the alphabet to refer to different steps to take.

Take some time each day, say 10 to 15 minutes in the beginning or end of the day, to prepare yourself for the following day—to remind yourself what you are going to be doing. You can also use this time to change anything around, such as determining that you need to reschedule an appointment because you have gotten too busy to make that meeting, and then you can send the person an e-mail to reschedule, leave a phone message, or call to speak to the person as convenient.

In short, don't only create a series of reminders, but regularly remind yourself about your reminders, too.

Then, with your reminder system in place, you can forget about the details until you have reminded yourself that you need to do so. The result? You have more of the mundane day-to-day details in these reminders, so you can free up your mind to focus on other activities that are more important to you. In other words, you will have to remember less, so you are better able to remember more!

11

Using Schemas and Scripts to Help You Remember

Another way to improve your memory is to incorporate what you learn or experience into a schema or script, though you have to be careful not to let these lead you into making faulty assumptions or stereotypes, which influence what you remember.

What Are Schemas and Scripts?

Essentially, a schema is your generalized knowledge about a situation or event, which leads you to expect things to be a certain way.[1] Additionally, you are likely to notice and remember things that fit your schema, and the reverse, to notice and remember things that are so unusual that they stand out.

For example, when you go to the grocery store, you have a schema for what the interior of the store looks like and what kind of objects and experiences to expect there. You expect the store to be laid out in aisles devoted to certain types of products; you expect the sales clerks to give you knowledgeable advice on where to go when you ask for directions; you expect to save money through certain types of savings programs; and so on. In turn, this schema helps you navigate the store as you become familiar with where things are. When there are changes, as when products are moved to another shelf or aisle, you may feel disoriented. Or you may feel annoyed if someone behaves in an unexpected way, such as if a clerk is short with you when you ask for directions, or if a clerk hovers too closely in giving you directions.

Schemas also help you remember new information, since they create a structure into which you can add related material. That's what helps experts better remember new material in their field; they incorporate it into a schema they already have. For instance, if you are a car enthusiast, you can easily remember details about new models and be able to distinguish them from other models. But someone who doesn't know about cars will find it hard to remember what's new and different about the latest model, much less compare it to other models. In fact, all sorts of cars may fuzz together in the novice's mind, so he or she can only remember broad distinctions, such as two-door, four-door; hard-top, convertible; sedan, convertible, station wagon, and SUV; and color. Likewise, if you don't know much about birds, you may only remember that you saw a small, dark bird on your porch yesterday, but someone who has studied about birds may pay attention to and remember such details as the bird's coloring, tail and wing formation, bill size, song if any, and even note its exact species and name.

Having a schema thus helps you fit new information into a structure of knowledge you already have. So you not only are more observant about what you see, but you can better encode that observation into that structure and therefore better remember.

As for scripts, these are a type of schema that features a simple, well-structured sequence of events in a specified order that you associate with a very familiar activity that occurs over a certain period of time,[2] like when you go to a restaurant. You go in, wait in line until the hostess seats you, then a waiter comes over to greet you, you look at the menu, you place your order, you have a conversation with the person you are with, eat your dinner, leave a tip, pull out a credit card, and sign for your bill.

How Schemas and Scripts Can Improve Your Memory

One way to use a schema or script for memory improvement is to consciously create a schema for acquiring new knowledge and remember the overall structure you have created. Then you can better incorporate new knowledge and therefore remember what you learn.

For example, when I first took a birding class, I didn't know very much about different types of birds. I just knew the names for familiar birds, like crows, robins, ostriches, parrots, and penguins. But I didn't know anything about the different families of birds, such as the categories for waterfowl (like geese, ducks, gulls, herons) or raptors, like hawks, falcons, kites, eagles, and vultures. However, rather than have us remember lists of different birds—over 100 common species in the California Bay Area alone—our instructor gave us an organizational method to use in which we should first look at the general characteristics of the bird, such as size of bird, bill size and shape, behavior, colors, songs and calls or other vocalizations, habitat, flight pattern, and how many birds are together. We used this information to identify the bird's family (e.g., owls), and then looked for more specific details to distinguish different types of owls, such as a barn owl, which is a small owl with a pale monkey face that looks something like an alien from another planet; a great horned owl, which is a large owl with ear tufts that look like the horns of a devil; and a burrowing owl, which is a small owl with long legs and ear tufts. This way, rather than having to remember all the birds individually, we could place them within a hierarchical structure for easier identification.

Structuring New Information into Categories to Create Your Own Schemas

As with my experience in the birding class, whenever you are learning new information, think about how you might structure it into overall categories; then fit the specific details into the categories with the best fit. In some cases, you may be taught these categories to help you learn and remember something; but if not, create your own categories so you better make sense of all this new information. Then, thinking of a category will trigger your memory of what's in the category.

This approach is a variation of the technique of creating hierarchies of categories, and it incorporates the important memory principle of chunking. Chunking is discussed in detail in Chapter 12, but in brief, it involves dividing information up into smaller, more memorable chunks, such as grouping between four and seven items together into one chunk, another four to seven items into another chunk, and so forth. But creating schemas with hierarchies takes the process of creating categories one step further, by organizing them into their own hierarchy of categories. Then, when you think of the category on top, that will help to trigger your memory for its subcategories, and as you focus on one of these subcategories, that will trigger your memory to think of the subcategories within that category, and so on, until you remember the more specific details.

Using a Schema to Remember What Happened

Having an overall schema for an event or experience can also help you remember what happened there, as you call up your schema and seek to reconstruct what happened, where, and when. For example, say you have a schema for going to a club with friends to listen to music. This schema may not be conscious for you, if you haven't thought about it before. But as you reflect on the overall experience, you may come up with your own series of common activities (i.e., you arrive, pay an entrance fee, go to the bar, take some drinks to the table, observe a series of acts perform, talk to your friends, dance, etc.).

One way this schema of what you generally do or your script for a particular evening can be especially useful is if you are trying to remember something later, such as where you were likely to have put down your keys. As you visualize the schema or script in your mind, you can see yourself as you go through different activities in order, rather than rushing around from place to place where you might have been. Just visualize in your mind going from one place to another in the order in which you normally do that activity. That way, you may recall where you placed the object and you can make a beeline to your lost object.

Or as you imagine the sequence mentally, go backwards to reconstruct the steps, so you remember the latest action, what you did before that, and so on, until you are back to where you were when you misplaced the item. However, when you do retrace your steps backwards, you may be calling on your logical mind to help you remember things in reverse order, which is harder to do. Generally, it is easier and more effective to simply go with the original flow. In fact, you may sometimes find what you are looking for without thinking about it—as if by calling up a script for a particular sequence of activities, you have tapped into the power of your unconscious mind. This will take you where you want to go as if you are on automatic, and voila, there are the keys, the cell phone, or whatever else you are looking for.

Calling up a schema or script might also help you more clearly remember particular conversations you had at a particular time. You literally see yourself having that conversation and that helps to trigger your memory of what was said.

Designing your own schema for something you have learned can also help you retain this information in your memory. One approach is to create an outline for the material, if you haven't already been given one, such as when you do an interview with someone and want to remember what was said. If you are taking notes at the time, you might jot down some trigger words to create the outline. If you are trying to remember later, focus on recalling the general topics first; then fit the details under those. You can create such an outline in a linear format (i.e., 1, 1a and 1b, 2, 2a, 2b, 2c, and so on).

You also can set up your outline in a graphic format so it becomes essentially a mind map, with subtopics branching off from the main topic, and then sub-subtopics branching off these. For example, a graphic outline might look something like this. Then, by remembering the main categories in the outline, you can better remember all of the details.

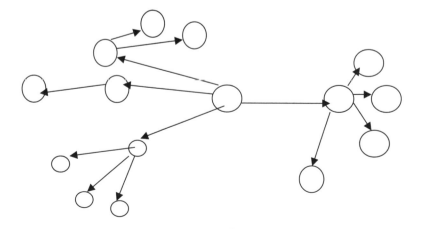

Practicing Sample Schemas and Scripts

To become familiar with using schemas and scripts, here are some common situations that make good examples to practice with. Remember, schemas are the more general patterns; scripts the more specific sequence that occurs over a particular time period. Use either one and see how vividly and concretely you can create your own schema or script.

- Going to the grocery store
- Eating out at a restaurant
- Going to a local dance or night club
- Visiting the zoo
- Preparing for and giving a presentation
- Shopping at a department store
- Attending or leading a staff meeting at work

As you visualize the usual sequence of activities, you can imagine what you have done in the past. Or you can project yourself into the future, so you imagine what to do to shape your future behavior. Then, when you are in the actual setting—when the future has become the present—you can tap into your memory of how you want to now behave, and so you are better able to do this. The process is a little like practicing a skill in your mind through mental imagery. If you practice the skill correctly, you will improve with the help of this mental imagery. However, the difference here is that instead of imagining a skill, you are imagining a whole experience.

This schema or script can also come in handy if someone wants you to recall what happened at an event, from your boss to a cop who is trying to elicit truthful testimony. The scenario will help you re-experience what happened, as you move around the scene and recall what occurred where. It is like you are seeing it now, using the schema or script in your mind.

Using Schemas for Better Recall

Using a schema can be a good way to recall information, particularly information that fits the schema, so you expect it to be there. For example, say you are reporting on an event or experience. If you remind yourself to pay close attention at the time and then later call up a visual image of what you observed, your schema (which includes your expectations of what is there) will give you mental triggers so you are able to remember in more detail. That's because of the process of selection, which leads you to more accurately recall information that is consistent with a particular schema—something that fits in, such as noticing and recalling calculators and record books on the desk of a bank officer.

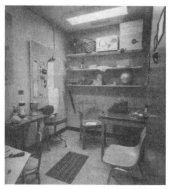

For example, two psychologists tried an experiment asking people to recall what they remembered about a psychologist's office where they were recently waiting for a few minutes. Most people remembered what was consistent with their schema for such an office—such as the desk and chair—but few remembered the unusual items—such as a wine bottle, coffee pot, and picnic basket—because these were inconsistent with the schema.[3]

Problems with Using Schemas and Scripts

One danger is that in trying to be consistent with your schema, you may recall things that weren't actually there, though you may think they were. For instance, in the experiment described above, about a half dozen participants remembered items that weren't in the room—such as books—because typically books would be in such an office.[4] It's the same reason why eyewitnesses in a criminal case might remember things that weren't there—such as thinking a person talking in a threatening manner was holding a gun—because it's consistent with their knowledge or expectations,.

Thus, while most of the time a schema can help you accurately retrieve information, there are times when you might feel certain you remembered something correctly, but in fact you were mistaken—because you are recalling things based on your prior knowledge and expectations, not what was actually there.

On the other hand, you may be more apt to notice and remember something that is very unusual, because it is inconsistent with an ordinary schema, such as when someone who is dressed inappropriately appears at an event. In such a situation, you may remember quite accurately, because you pay closer attention, since you have been jarred out of operating on automatic—the way you more typically record everyday schemas that fit your usual expectations.

Another time for caution is when you try to recall conversations because of a memory process that psychologists call "abstraction," where you store what the message means but not the exact words or sentence structure.[5] You may think you have recalled a conversation correctly, but commonly you store the gist of the message or its general meaning. Another source of error is that you might combine various facts together in your memory. Once you do this, you cannot separate them into what you originally heard or observed, so you can't recall exactly the original.[6] This phenomenon of not being able to distinguish thoughts from what you actually experienced might be particularly important when you are claiming you had a verbal agreement with someone and you each remember that agreement differently. This is a good reason to write any agreement down and not leave it to memory; your memory could be wrong, just as the other party's could be, but you each are equally certain that you are right.

A way to counteract this source of memory error is to pay careful attention to the exact words in a particular sentence, since you can strategically control your attention. When you do pay close attention, psychologists have found, your memory can be quite accurate.[7] Obviously, this kind of attention isn't merited for everything you hear; it would be mentally overtaxing to try to continually focus your attention on everything. But if you selectively pick out what you want to attend to more closely, you will be able to remember that.

As an exercise, try carefully paying attention to something you hear or read. To be able to check your accuracy, record what you hear on a tape recorder or cassette recorder so you can play it back. Then, work on remembering a sentence and afterwards listen to the tape again or look at what was written. Count how many words out of the total you got right and divide the total words by that number to get a percentage score. You will find your percentages will be higher for shorter sentences, lower for longer ones. But as you practice paying attention and remembering, your percentages reflecting your ability to remember should increase.

Try testing yourself with shorter sentences (i.e., 5–10 words) first; then try longer sentences (i.e., 11–15 words); and then still longer ones (i.e., 16–20 words). You will find that your percentages should increase for each category. As for the usual guideline about only being able to remember seven plus or minus two items (the "Magic Number Seven," discussed in Chapter 1), you can remember more when you are working with sentences, because they have meaning and you also have grammatical rules to guide you—essentially a language schema that helps you remember meaningful sentences that make sense to you.

Another caution is about remembering inferences or logical interpretations and conclusions that were not part of the original information you received. This can occur because your own interests and background can shape what you remember; they can also lead you to add additional information to what you have seen or heard.[8] Then, too, you may use a process known as "reconstruction" to fill in missing details based on your expectations about what should be there. For example, you may recall who was in a staff meeting and think that one person who is normally there was present, when, in fact, that person wasn't there on that day. In everyday life, such reconstructions often are correct, but not always.

Do you remember the classic game of "rumor" (sometimes called "telephone"), which you probably played during your childhood? One person starts the rumor by whispering a sentence or two to the next person in line; that person repeats the message to the next person; and so on down the line, until the last person announces aloud what he or she heard. Then the first person says what he or she said in the beginning. Usually, there is a great difference between what was originally stated and what the last person says, resulting in much hilarity.

Well, the same thing can happen in everyday life, such as when one person shares a story over the water cooler and another person hears it and passes it on. Typically, what happens is that each person will recall the gist of the story and may then add his or her own additional information and inferences in telling the story to the next person, who will then do the same in passing the story on. So what may start out as a simple statement that an employee is leaving the company may turn into a drama about how that employee is leaving because he or she doesn't like working there and had a fight with the boss.

To experiment with this process, get a few friends or business associates together and use the structure of the game of rumor, except instead of just a sentence or two, take about a minute to start a story with some details. Include information about the person's job, work activities, and an incident that occurs affecting that person and others in the company. Record what you have stated, so you are able to play it back at the end. Then, the next person similarly tells the story to another person, trying to capture the same kind of drama and detail as in the story they heard. Finally, at the end, the last person tells the story to the whole group. After that, replay the original story, and notice the differences. What got conveyed accurately? What got changed? What kind of additional information was added? What was added that was consistent with the original story? What was added that was inconsistent, but may reflect the experiences and outlook of someone in the group who added that information?

In short, use your experience with telling the story to help you better understand your own memory processes and those of others in using schemas and scripts.

12

Chunk It and Categorize It

Chunking is one of a number of organizational principles to help you more effectively encode information by putting it into a series of smaller packages that are easier to remember. One way to do this is to simply break up the information. In addition, you can further organize it into clusters or hierarchical categories, and when you call up the clusters or categories, you will better remember what you put in them. It's like putting your CD collection into categories by genre.

Another approach is to combine chunking with using imagery to remember different chunks, as described in Chapter 20, or to combine the chunks into a story or narrative, as described in Chapter 16). Plus you can use rehearsal (Chapter 13) to further reinforce what you have chunked or grouped into categories.

In short, think of chunking and clustering or organizing information into categories as two types of tools that you can use in combination with other tools to reinforce your memory.

How Chunking and Categorizing Works

In chunking you combine several smaller units—whether they are numbers, names, places, objects, or anything—into larger units. You can take them in the order they are already in or combine them into clusters or categories, sometimes called a hierarchy, according to some organizing principle, such as names beginning with a certain letter, age groups, region of the country, or types of animals. The reason this kind of organization is called a hierarchy is that the group or category you have put individual items into is considered a higher order category. In fact, if you have a number of categories, you can further chunk them into groups and put those in even higher order categories.

You might visualize this hierarchy in a graphic form, such as in the chart below.

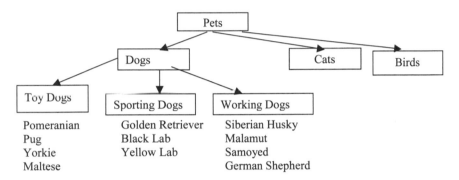

Or you can organize the hierarchy into an outline with topics and subtopics. While a graphic is good when you are trying to remember words, phrases, names, objects, and other small bits of information, an outline is good when you are learning concepts or more complex information. In either case, you encode the information in the chunks and organizational structures you have created. Later, when you seek to retrieve the memory, tapping into the category of information you want will help you pull out the information in that category. Think of the process as putting information in a file cabinet and creating files for information and categories for where you want to file information. You don't have to look through all of the loose papers or files to find what you want; the organizational system you created will help you get there quickly.

As researchers have found in repeated tests, people recall more information when it is grouped into more familiar, meaningful categories than placed into an arbitrary group of information.[1]

Get Chunky with It

Here are some examples of how plain vanilla chunking works. Often you will get numbers given to you that are already chunked up, such as phone numbers, which are usually in three chunks (e.g., 510-123-4569), and bank accounts in two or three chunks (e.g., 423-912-776 or 23455-40544). But sometimes you will get other numbers or number and letter combinations that are just *loooong*, such as a password or registration number for software that has been assigned to you. While using a memory support (such as a file for important numbers and passwords, as discussed in Chapter 10) may be helpful, since you then don't have to remember such numbers, there may be times you want to remember them.

For example, you may want to keep the combination for a lock in your memory as well as in a security deposit box for security reasons and convenience; you may need a password when you use a different computer and don't immediately have access to your password file. While paying careful attention and occasional rehearsal may help implant these numbers and letters in your memory, chunking will make the process far easier.

For example, suppose you have a list of numbers, such as: 19141492196317761890200011942.

Try glancing at it for a minute or two without trying to do any chunking. Then, without looking at the numbers, on a separate piece of paper write down as many numbers as you can in sequence.

Did you find it hard to do? How far did you get? Normally, you will not be able to remember more than four or five numbers.

Now, look back at the numbers and think about how you might chunk them up into bits that are easier to remember. Do you notice anything yet that will help you remember?

If you didn't already get it, think dates, and break up the numbers accordingly:

1914 1492 1963 1776 1890 2001 1942

Now close the book again, take another minute, try to remember them in sequence, and see how far you get.

Finally, you might further organize the dates chronologically, which will serve as another aid to memory. Try to remember this new list of numbers (I changed the dates, since you will already be primed from the previous test: 1512178918651920194619722003. Again, close the book, take a minute, and see how many you remembered now. Again, compare your results from the first and second tests, and you should see some improvement: 1512 1789 1865 1920 1946 1972 2003.

To make the dates stand out even more, you might combine the dates with visual associates, since it's easier to remember these. If the date is well known, such as 1865, the beginning of the Civil War, you can combine that with an image of Civil War soldiers in battle. But if it's just a random date, you might associate it with some image from the general period, such as associating a peasant in the field with 1512.

Here's a similar experiment to try with letters. See how far you get in remembering the letters in each condition. Don't look at the next set until you have tested yourself on the first one.

1. A list: ATLNASACIANBCACLULAX

2. A chunked list: ATL NASA CIA NBC ACLU LAX

3. An alphabetized chunked list (again, I have changed the items):
   AMA BBC FBI INTEL NYC SONY

Or suppose you just have a list of numbers, letters, or numbers and letters that don't form a real word when you chunk them. You can still do better by chunking them and trying to remember each group than by trying to remember everything in the list.

For example, try the following sets of letters or numbers without chunking them and see how far you get. As before, study each list for about a minute, close the book, and write down the letters or numbers in sequence on a sheet of paper. (You can also generate your own lists to experiment with by randomly writing down a series of numbers, letters, or numbers and letters. Then proceed as with the lists in the book or swap lists with a friend or associate who is working on developing his or her memory.) I have created lists with 12 to 16 letters or numbers. You can make your own lists longer or shorter than this as you experiment with how much you can remember.

Just Letters: RBYAWPOQNMIEUYRY
AURPWUNFGSLF

Just Numbers: 1746039758942875
385019843873

Letters and Numbers: 27G89T34097R238W
G589Y34N893T

Now try chunking these into groups and see how many you can remember. I've suggested one way to chunk these into groups of four letters or numbers, but you can chunk these in other groups—say three or four letters or numbers as you prefer.

Just Letters: RBYA WPOQ NMIE UYRY
AURP WUNF GSLF

Just Numbers: 1746 0397 5894 2875
3850 1984 3873

Letters and Numbers: 27G8 9T34 097R 238W
G589 Y34N 893T

Creating Categories and Groups

You've already seen some examples of creating categories and groups in the discussion of how this process works, and you've done some simple grouping with letters and numbers. Now I'll discuss different ways of creating the categories yourself, so you come up with an optimal way of grouping information that works well for you.

Some possible ways of grouping information include basing them on:

- Formal categories for types (such as based on type of animal, group of dog, breed of dog)
- Characteristics of the word (such as first letter, length of word, rhyming)
- Meaning of topic

- Priority or your interest in the subject
- Visual characteristics (such as objects that are round, square, oval)

To demonstrate the power of creating categories, try the exercises in the following section. First, you will see some lists of randomly organized words or topics. Take a minute or two to remember the items in the first list, close the book, and write down as many items as you can recall. Then, take the words or items in the second list, which is grouped into categories, take a minute to remember the words, and see how many you remember. Generally, you should be able to remember more words in the second list.

Then, apply this creating categories technique whenever you have a list of items to remember—such as a grocery list or names of stores to visit in a shopping center.

You can create your own lists of words and topics to further experiment with this technique. Work with a partner or in a group, where one party comes up with a list of words or topics that are listed randomly or included in categories. Then, the other party has to look at the list for a minute, turn it over, and see how many he or she can recall in a minute or two.

Creating Categories with Words

Following are three recall tests with several sets of words. Take a minute to look at the words in each set in turn, look away from the book, and write down as many as you can. The words don't have to be in a sequence. After you create your list, see how many you can recall under each of the conditions mentioned below.

I have used different but similar words in each set, so your memory from a previous test will not carry over to the next test. You can similarly create lists and categories in working with a partner or group for all of these tests.

Recall Test 1: Word, Words, Words

Here's a list of words in no particular order. Remember as many as you can in 1 minute. Then see how many you can recall correctly, and write down your score, 1 point for each.

Cat

Lettuce

Fish

Store

Clock

Parrot

Printer

Box

Monitor

Factory

Nation

Newspaper

Bell

Telephone

Dance

Window

Recall Test 2: Words in Categories

This is one possible way of organizing words into categories.

Animals	Equipment	Shopping	Work
Dog	Computer	Grocery	Office
Turtle	Lamp	Counter	Package
Eagle	Desk	Cash	Fax
	Bookshelf	Milk	Project
		Pizza	

Recall Test 3: You Create the Categories

As you look at these words, create your own categories to help trigger your memory.

Baseball

Watch

Refrigerator

Teller

Television

Guitar

Football

Fox

Furnace

Tiger

Shoe

Bank

Movie

Piano

Raccoon

Now let's try two recognition tests. Your task is to pick out from the second list those words that were in the first list, under each of these conditions: (1) when you only see a list of words, (2) when you see the words in a group. Then, compare your results. You should find your ability goes up when you use categories. The process should also help you quickly come up with and remember categories to use in grouping lists of anything you want to learn in the future.

Recognition Test #1: Is It a Match?

Without using any categories, study List #1 for 1 minute. Next, without looking at the first list, make a checkmark next to each word in List #2 that appeared in List #1. Then, look back at List #1 and compare. Score 1 point for each correct match; also score 1 point for each unchecked word that was *not* in List #1. Deduct 1 point for every incorrect answer.

List #1	List #2
	Cover Up Until Ready For Test
Snail	House
Wire	Mile
Mouse	Honey
Baggage	Roof
Poem	Candle
Red	Red
Mirror	Flower

Oven	Car
Mile	Turkey
Jazz	Train
Bucket	Sink
Flower	Music
Car	Cat
Green	Trick
Honey	Donkey
Candle	Poem

Recognition Test #2: Group Game

Now test your memory when you have categories for placing the items you want to remember. Afterwards, compare the results with your previous recall results.

List #1		List #2
		Cover Up Until Ready For Test
Animals:	Horse	Chin
	Cow	Compact
	Snake	Bicycle
Parts of the Body:	Chin	Dress
	Eye	Clerk
	Foot	Bus
Types of Vehicles:	Compact	Bull
	Van	Soap
	Bus	Monster
Shopping:	Dress	Cashier
	Curtain	Face
	Soap	Boss
	Perfume	Shark
	Party	Eye
Work:	Boss	Tower
	Clerk	Plane

Creating and Using Categories in Your Work and Personal Life

Now that you've seen the power of using categories to remember more, here are some ways you might use categories to remember different types of things.

- Create a more organized shopping list, where you categorize everything on your list by the type of product. Then, review these items before you go shopping, and you can better remember what you need to get. You might even organize your list according to the aisles in your grocery store, so you can zoom down the aisles getting what you need. You can do it much faster, since you don't have to continually look at your list. It'll all be in your head, and as you go down each aisle, that will trigger what's in a particular category. (You should probably check your list before you get to the checkout counter, just to be on the safe side.)

- Organize a talk or presentation with an outline; then prepare by memorizing the sequence of the main categories of the outline first. Once you have those down solid, work on remembering the items in each category. (You'll find more tips for how to apply other techniques to better remember what you are going to say or present in Chapter 29.)

- Organize the material in a course you are studying into an outline (if you haven't already been given an outline for the class). Then, as in organizing your own talk or presentation, focus on learning the main categories first, and then use that as a trigger to help you remember what is in each section. After that you can use other techniques like chunking and highlighting keywords to trigger a more detailed memory for different points you want to remember.

- Organize products, types of services, or types of activities into categories to help you remember to talk about them—a great aid if you are in sales or teaching. If you have a table of contents or outline that already does this, use it as a guide—but don't just read it straight through. Learn each of the categories first and then the information within it. Or create your own outline. Then, within each category, prioritize what's most important to talk about first, and focus on encoding that into your memory first. In effect, you are creating an organizational schema that will facilitate your putting additional memories into that schema.

• Organize the business cards of people you meet into categories, such as type of business, to help you in remembering the names of all these people. Then, review these cards by category, and to help you further remember, organize them alphabetically or prioritize those that are most important to remember. Again, the categories form a schema to help you recall the names—plus you can use other memory aids to be discussed in the next few chapters and in Chapter 27 to further flesh out your memory of each person.

So what other types of lists or collections of information do you want to remember? Where appropriate, create categories to help you remember, in addition to any other memory techniques you use.

13

Rehearse . . . Rehearse . . . Rehearse . . . and Review

Unless you are one of the rare individuals with a photographic or eidetic memory, you generally have to review what you have learned, sometimes several times, to fully implant the new learning in your memory. Later, if you have been away from the material for awhile, you have to review it again to refresh the memory; you need the repetition to remember.

I have frequently heard it said in classes and workshops that you forget about 70 percent of what you have learned in one day and after a few days, it's about 90 percent. But you can increase what you remember when you learn using multiple models of encoding, since the encoding uses multiple memory traces.

You've probably had some of these experiences more than once:

- You've seen a great movie, but a few days later, you only have a fuzzy idea of the plot and may not even be able to remember the name of the movie without prompting.

- You read a book about current trends and are very impressed with the expertise of the writer. But later that week, when someone asks you what impressed you so much about the writer's argument, you can't remember what he said any-

145

more—you only have a general impression that it was a great book.

- You go to a classroom lecture and take copious notes, but when you look at your notes a couple of weeks later to study for the exam, you don't even recognize what you wrote.
- You have collected a set of business cards at a networking event. When you look at them several days later, you don't have the slightest idea who most of the names are and can barely remember what you talked about with the people you do remember.

Such forgetting is common—it's our way of coping with the flood of information we get each day. This daily deluge includes not only the information you'd like to remember but the things you'd like to forget (like the annoying commercials you watched during the commercial breaks, since you didn't feel like getting up for a couple of minutes to do something else).

So when you do want to remember something, review and rehearsal can help you solidify the memory in your mind. You can use other recall techniques too, since this process is apart from anything else you do to enter the information in your memory (such as chunking, imagery associations, using trigger words, and the all about me principle). In review, you go over what you have just learned to more firmly encode it in the first place; in rehearsal, you expand on your initial review with a return to the material, so you firmly fix that encoding in place. It's like what an actor does to learn his or her part in a script—the first reading is like a review; then the actor goes over and over it on his or her own, followed by more extensive rehearsals with a group of other actors. The result: a flawless performance on stage or a minimal number of takes for a film.

The process can be applied to all sorts of memory tasks:

- Recalling the names of people you have met at a networking event or conference.
- Reviewing your notes from a class or a meeting.
- Remembering what you have written in your daily calendar for the next few days.

- Giving a speech or presentation.
- You name it.

Using the Review Process Effectively

A good way to use the review process is to go over whatever you have written down or collected soon after you have initially recorded or collected this information. If you are giving a speech or presentation, write down an outline for what you plan to say, and review that. When you do your review, add any relevant notes to help trigger your memory later—or use brackets, underlines, or a highlighter to point up what you want to remember. You might also underline or circle certain trigger words.

The advantage of doing this review process sooner rather than later is that you will be more familiar with this material (remember, we forget 90 percent of what we have learned after a few days), so you will better understand what your notes or the materials you have collected are all about. If you have taken extensively detailed notes or written down trigger words at the time (such as noting why you are collecting certain business cards at the time), you can generally skip this initial review step. That's because your notes or notations will be complete enough so you will know what this is all about later. But otherwise, do this review soon after you have initially taken the notes or collected materials, so you aren't later puzzled by your notes, collected cards, or other materials you don't understand.

You obviously don't want to take the time to do a review for something you are doing for recreation, such as reading a novel. In that case, it doesn't matter if you forget the information. But for anything you need to know for work or school, take the extra time to do this.

For example, here's what I've been doing for the initial review for classes I've been taking in Anthropology, Mass Communications and Organizational/Consumer/Audience Behavior, and Pop Culture and Lifestyles. Since I have learned to take very detailed notes, I usually wait to do the review a few days before any test or discussion about the material. At this time, I bracket what I feel is most important, since this is what I will focus on in the additional review or rehearsal phase.

As for business cards, if I have made notes on the cards, so I know what to do with them, I skip the review process. Otherwise, I go over the cards and either put them into piles of cards with notes on what to do with that group of cards (such as telling my assistant to add their names to a database with a code for their area of interest and source where I have gotten the card) or I write down a notation on that card about what to do with that card for follow-up later.

Rehearsing to Get It Right

After you do an initial review, rehearse at least once more with this material to solidify the information in your memory. As you work more often with this process, you will find how much rehearsal you need to do for different types of material. As a general rule, the more material you have, the more you need to rehearse in order to remember it all. If you are giving a speech, presentation, or other kind of performance, you can either gather the content and create an outline for this—or come up with an outline and fill in the content. But in either case, go over the outline so you have that firmly implanted in your mind, since that will provide a trigger for the content in that section. Then, once you have the content firmly in memory, you can add the dramatic flair you want for your final program.

The process is a little bit like what actors have to do in preparing for a scene in a film or a stage play. If the actor only has a few lines, a couple of individual rehearsals may be all that's needed to encode the lines into memory before the actor goes through the lines in a group rehearsal. But if the actor has a much longer scene to prepare for, more rehearsal is necessary. If it's a full stage play, particularly a leading part, even more rehearsal time is needed.

It's best to time your rehearsal for a few days or even a night before you have to know the material. If you are going to be doing more than one rehearsal, it's best to space it over two or three days, rather than trying to have two rehearsals on the same day. That's because, as previously discussed, the unconscious processes that occur while you are sleeping help to consolidate what you have learned in your memory.

Once you have determined the number of rehearsals that work for you for different types and amounts of memory tasks, use that as a guide in the future when you have other things to learn and commit to memory. Later, as your memory improves, you may find you need fewer rehearsals. Why? Because you are encoding the material in more detail, particularly if you are combining rehearsal with other memory techniques. Also, as you learn material in a particular field, you are creating a schema in your mind that facilitates learning other material that fits within this schema. (See Chapter 11 for more discussion about creating schemas and scripts.)

For example, after some experimentation, I have found that the following process works well for me in learning new material:

1. An initial review of my detailed notes and any articles or books a few days before a presentation or exam, which includes bracketing or highlighting the sections of special interest, and underlining important trigger words.
2. A second reading of these materials, paying special attention to the items I have bracketed and the words I have highlighted.
3. A third review of the items I have bracketed and the words I have highlighted; this should take place the night before—or even the morning of—the scheduled exam, discussion, presentation, etc.

Find out what works for you by experimenting to determine how much rehearsal you need for different types and amounts of information. Then, if you are presenting or performing this material, add in additional rehearsal time to practice, practice, practice, so you remember all the extra dramatic touches to make your performance shine.

Reviewing and Rehearsing with Others

Besides reviewing and rehearsing on your own, you can also engage in these activities with others to further stimulate your ability to remember through the reinforcement and support that others provide. Plus it can be fun to engage in these memory activities with others. This combination of reinforcement, support, and fun is the reason why many students create study groups at school—both to learn the material in the first place or to go over and recall it later.

If you do get together with a group, keep the group small, so everyone gets to participate—three or four people is ideal, and limit the group to no more than five or six people. You can always split into two smaller groups if the group gets too large.

Find a comfortable place you can meet that is free of distractions. Turn off your cell phones; right now, you are unavailable. After brief preliminary socializing is out of the way, focus on what you want to learn and remember. A good approach is to have participants summarize in turn the major points they have gotten from the material. Or have the first person do the summary, and then each person in turn adds something new. After everyone has had a chance to summarize or add to the summary, the first person to start a round of summarizing does a brief recap.

As others speak, take notes if you wish on your material or on a separate sheet of paper to highlight especially important points to remember. Later, you can rehearse the material and what you have learned from the group review or rehearsal on your own. The advantage of the group process is that it adds to the multi-model memory channels, since you are encoding your experience of the group process along with your own performance of the material, in addition to the content of the material.

Increasing Your Review and Rehearsal Power

To increase your encoding and retrieval ability at both the review and rehearsal stage, combine these processes with other memory techniques. This way, when you review and rehearse, you have a more detailed and solid memory, because you are using multiple memory channels. In particular, here's how these other techniques can help.

- Use the all about me principle to think about whatever you are initially encoding into memory to highlight why this is impor-

tant to you. Then, when you rehearse, you might remind yourself why this is important to you.

- Use chunking to group different sections of what you want to
  remember together, such as if you have identified a series of
  trigger words in a speech, article, or book chapter. Then, pay
  attention to these groupings and where different items of information fit as you review and rehearse the material.

- Use imagery associations, so as you review and rehearse, you
  see a picture in your mind to reinforce what you are taking in
  verbally. Or in some cases, experience yourself in the scene of
  whatever you are reading or hearing about, which is particularly helpful if you are reading a narrative.

- Use a group discussion to further reinforce what you have
  learned.

- Plus use any other memory techniques that are applicable to
  the material you are trying to remember.

Putting Review and Rehearsal into Practice

How much review and rehearsal do you need for different things you
are learning? Try experimenting with different types of material to
find out.

A good way to start is with a short article, chapter in a book, or
section of a talk you are going to give. Go over it once for an initial
review, making brackets, notes, or underlining trigger words.

Then, imagine that you are describing what you have just re-
viewed to someone else and, mentally or speaking aloud, state the
highlights of this material. After you do this, notice how much you
have remembered. Have you been able to remember details? Or do
you only recall the vague gist of what the material is about? Briefly
write down your reflections about your experience.

Now, do a first rehearsal of this material—or take a similar article, chapter, or section of a talk, and do a review and then a rehearsal. During this rehearsal, as described above, quickly review all
the material, but pay particular attention to any of the material you
have bracketed, any trigger words, and anything you have noted.
After you do this, repeat the imaginary retelling, as described above,

to see how much you have remembered. Ask yourself if you have been able to remember details or just the vague gist of what the material is about. Compare your experience with this first rehearsal and your initial review. Did you recall more detail? Briefly write down your reflections about your experience.

Then, do a second rehearsal of this material—or take a similar article, chapter, or section of a talk, and do a review, first rehearsal, and second rehearsal. Use the same process as described above to determine your recall.

Generally, you will find that with each rehearsal, your memory of the material becomes stronger and stronger.

As you rehearse longer or different material, notice how this experience compares to using the process with shorter material. Increase the rehearsal time as needed for longer and more complex material, depending on how well you need to know the details. For example, sometimes you just need to know the general concepts and principles described in an article or chapter; in other cases, you need the details, such as examples or stories illustrating these principles. Adapt how much you have to rehearse as you learn more about your own memory processes. Working with these processes will help you get a better sense of how much rehearsal you need depending on the type of material, its length, and how much detail you need to know.

14

Repeat It!

A close cousin of rehearsal is simply repeating something as you hear it, and in some cases, embellishing it with another technique, such as using imagery or making other types of associations. The difference is that the rehearsal technique described in the previous chapter is for longer, more complex information where you are trying to remember more details. Repetition is a way to remember simpler bits of information, such as names of people, phone and bank account numbers, and street directions. You are not so much reviewing and rehearsing this information as repeating it over and over to drum it into your memory.

A classic example of how this works is the old memory game that many kids learn at school or camp to remember names—and sometimes adults play, too. Everyone sits in a circle or group. In turn, each person says their name and the names in order of every person who previously said their name. Players keep going until someone misses a name; then that person is out and the next player continues from there. The last person left in the game is declared the winner. For example:

- The first player says TED.
- The second player says TED and his own name, JERRY.
- The third player says TED and JERRY and her own name, SUSIE.

• The fourth player says TED, JERRY, SUSIE, and her own name, JILL.

And so on. The game is typically used as an icebreaker, and the usual outcome is that everyone knows and remembers everyone else's name, since they learned this through repetition.

The process of repetition is one you can use for almost anything because we think faster than we listen to something.

Using Repetition in Everyday Life

When you use repetition, pick out what's important to you; you obviously don't want to go around repeating everything to yourself. For example, if you are introduced to a large number of people during the evening, it might be better to collect cards from everyone where possible and use repetition for the names of the people whom you want to talk with further. (See Chapter 27, which is devoted specifically to remembering names and faces.) Also, as you repeat something, use images or associations to make it even more vivid to you. If you have a number of things to remember at one time, like a series of numbers for an account or a password, use chunking, too, to make what you repeat to yourself even easier. (Chapter 28 is devoted to remembering numbers.)

Consider using either mental or physical repetition, or both. For mental repetition, use self-talk to say the person's name over and over to yourself. For physical repetition, say the person's name out loud or write it down, using it in a context that makes sense, such as by prefacing a statement or question with the person's name or giving a reason why you are writing the person's name down, such as "I want to contact you later about this program we talked about."

Here are some examples from everyday life of how you might use repetition.

1. You meet someone and want to remember that person's **name.** Say that person's name over several times in your mind; then make a comment to that person using his or her name, such as "That's an interesting point you are making, **Henry.**" At the same

time, you might reinforce repeating the name mentally and physically with an image, such as seeing a clucking **hen**, which will become an image association with Henry. Or use the all about me method to think about how you might work with Henry in the future or how a relationship with Henry might benefit you.

2. You listen to a lecture and want to remember an **idea** that was expressed. (This is not to be confused with trying to remember extensive details about this lecture, as described in Chapter 13.) State the idea to yourself mentally and repeat that statement several more times to yourself. Then, if you want to embed it even more firmly, use the all about me approach to think about how you can further gain from this idea—or for a negative idea, how you can avoid the consequences.

3. You hear or see a **phone number, bank account number,** or **password** and want to remember it. In this case, you may already have a place where you have written this information down—a good idea, because you don't want to keep a lot of numbers in your head that can fade over time. But for convenience, you want to access these numbers quickly, too. Ideally, slow down the pace of learning these numbers, so you can repeat each number to yourself without interference from another number. Then, for each number, if it isn't already chunked, chunk it up, and mentally repeat that number to yourself. Additionally, to help remember what each number is for, create an image for that item or organization. For instance, if it's a phone number, visualize the image of a phone next to the number. If it's a bank account, visualize the bank where you have the account. If it's a password, create an image for the Website or account where it is a password, such as imagining a camera for a site featuring films or a newspaper for a daily news site. You can use your memory of real images, humorous cartoon images, company logos, or whatever helps to make the link between the number to remember and the place where you can use it.

4. You are getting **directions** about somewhere you need to go. For security, it is best to actually write these down if you have more than three or four steps to remember, because once you make a mistake like turning left instead of going right, you may get lost. But it's

often very convenient if you can remember these directions and not have to constantly look at what you have written—which can not only slow you down but cause an accident if you are driving in a car. To remember the directions, repeat the street or which way to go on it mentally to yourself as the person says it ("Turn right when you get to Maple Avenue" can become "right onto Maple"). At the same time, try to envision a map in your head, so you visually create a mental map to follow along with your mental soundtrack. You might also add in image associations as you hear each street name, such as seeing the image of a peach for Peachtree Lane, the image of a small mechanical gadget for Widget Road. As for the directions, as you say left, right, or straight ahead to yourself, you might see the image of an arrow on a street sign pointing in that direction. As for the distances, such as if someone tells you to go two blocks or go six miles, repeat those numbers to yourself, too. In Chapter 28, you will also learn to create associations with those numbers using the Number Shapes method, such as a "stick" for 1 or a "swan" for 2. See those images appear as you say the numbers.

5. You hear the **title** of a song, book, or movie or see it in print, on a Website, or on a movie marquee. Repeat the title to yourself several times—and again, it helps to think of an image you associate with the meaning of the words, for example, the image of a man behind bars while a bright red heart flashes above him for a song entitled "Guilty for Loving You."

Practice What You Repeat

Now that you've got the basic idea, concentrate on picking out things to repeat to yourself as you go through the day. At the same time, combine saying the words to yourself with using other memory reinforcers like the all about me or imagery associations techniques.

After you have used this technique for a few hours or a day, reflect on how well it has worked for you. To do so, think about each type of thing you have tried to remember (e.g., names at an event, ideas you have heard, phone or bank numbers, or directions) and see how well you recall it. You can do this mentally, or to further check yourself, write down the names, ideas, numbers, directions, or other items you have tried to remember through repetition. Compare what you've written to the real items and see how accurate you were. Determine the percentage of correct items remembered.

Do this exercise again and again over the next few days with new material, and compare your performance each day. You should find that for equivalent-sized lists, your percentages will go up. If you try this with a significantly larger list, your percentages will be likely to go down, since you have much more to remember. Conversely, with a significantly shorter list, your percentages should go up, because you have much less to remember. So for comparability, keep what you try to recall each day about the same amount.

15

Talk About It

As the proverbial "they" often say, if you want to really learn something, teach it. That goes for describing, explaining, and discussing it, too. So another way to firmly remember something is to describe it, explain it, discuss it, or teach it.

Think back to the times when you have been in a classroom or group discussion of some subject. You've read a book or article or seen a film or TV show that is up for discussion, and as you talk about it—particularly if you are the one doing the talking—you find you remember more. In fact, you may discover that you can remember much more than you originally thought you could, because as you talk about the subject, you trigger additional memories.

The same thing often happens when the police are talking to witnesses. As the witnesses are asked to describe more details about the incident they observed, what they say becomes clearer and more detailed in their mind. (Of course, you have to be careful about responding to leading questions, where a cop or a lawyer can actually put the details into your head. But as long as the questions are phrased in a general way to elicit more details from you—not suggest details *to* you—as you describe what you observed, you will see more.)

Thus, look for opportunities to describe and discuss with others something you want to remember, such as an experience you had or something you read or learned about. You also can imagine yourself doing an activity in your mind or you can perform in front of a mirror or recite into a tape recorder. You can use visualizations to help you as you describe, explain, discuss, or teach something. This technique also works well when combined with the all about me approach. Think about how this material is meaningful for you, not only for you personally, but how it might affect your community or society, and thereby impact on you as well.

Talk-About-It Techniques

Here are some techniques you can use to describe, explain, discuss, or teach to remember in different ways.

Just Tell It

Here you report on what you experienced to friends, family members, or associates who are willing listeners. You can describe or explain to an individual or to a group of people. As you do, make your account as vivid and interesting as possible. If you get any questions, answer them as completely as possible.

If you don't have a willing listener you can talk to, *imagine* you are telling someone. Imagine the person sitting in front of you, and talk to that person just as you would to a real person. Or if you prefer, imagine you are talking to a group of people. Preferably speak aloud, since this will help to further reinforce your memory, since you are speaking and using an auditory channel. But you can also do this mentally using both self-talk and visualizing yourself speaking to a person or group in your mind.

Mirror, Mirror

As an alternative to describing or explaining to a real or imaginary person or group, stand or sit in front of a mirror and describe or explain what you want to remember while you look in the mirror. Again, you can either speak aloud or imagine yourself speaking in your mind.

In this case, since there is no one else to ask questions, you can ask them yourself to create a dialogue and expand on your description or explanation. For instance, ask yourself questions like: "What else did you notice?" or "Can you explain more about how that happened?"

Be an Announcer

In this technique, imagine that you are an announcer on a TV show or radio program describing or explaining whatever you want to remember—from events and experiences to books, articles, films, TV shows, and lectures. Whatever it is, imagine that you are reporting on this as a news story, and as such, want to make it as dramatic and exciting as possible. For instance, you might start your description or explanation with a comment like: "And now this just in. Here's some breaking news . . ." Then, go into your account.

Again, you can do this announcer technique either with a willing audience or you can imagine an audience seated before you, as you play announcer in your home or office. Then, speak aloud or imagine yourself speaking in your mind. While speaking aloud is preferable to make the experience more powerful for you, discretion may be the better part of valor: You don't want to practice aloud if the people nearby are going to think you're nuts.

Discuss It

Here you want to get a dialogue going, such as with a group that has either experienced the same event or has read or viewed the same material. The back and forth will help to not only imprint the original information on your mind, but you'll have the reinforcement from the discussion and comments by others.

Alternatively, if you aren't able to discuss things with someone else or in a group, use your imagination to create a discussion. Imagine that you are in a group or in a dialogue with someone sitting before you and have the discussion with this imaginary individual or group. As you do, you can go back and forth, stating your ideas as you then agree, amplify, question, or challenge, speaking as another person. Or imagine this discussion going on in your mind, where you are speaking first as you and then as another person.

Teach It

Teaching is another great way to really learn and remember something. If you really are a teacher, you may, of course, be able to bring in something to teach and discuss, if it fits the subject matter of your class. Or if you can play the role of teacher in front of another person or a group, great! If you wish, invite questions and answer as completely as you can.

Otherwise, imagine you are a teacher, much as you might imagine being an announcer in the technique described above. Whatever you want to remember, imagine that you are in front of a class, teaching your students about what you have just learned. You can imagine yourself doing a demonstration to further illustrate what you are teaching in a more dramatic way. You can also imagine that your students are asking you questions, and then answer them.

While it is preferable to speak aloud to make the experience more powerful as in the announcer technique, you can also do this in your mind. Just see yourself playing the teacher, including doing demonstrations, asking for questions from students, and answering them—all in your mind's eye.

Putting These Techniques into Practice

Try experimenting with these different techniques in different formats—interacting in reality with others, imagining that you are interacting with others and speaking aloud, and visualizing your presentation and any interaction only in your mind. Then, notice what technique you prefer for remembering different types of information and rate how well you think you remembered what you were trying to describe, explain, discuss, or teach.

For example, you may prefer the "just tell it" approach for describing an experience, the "announcer" approach for talking about something you learned in the news, the "teacher" technique for something your read about, and so on. You should find that over time, your ability to describe, explain, discuss, or teach about something helps you remember details even more completely.

Use the chart on the following page to help you rate how well you are doing in using these different techniques for different purposes and in different formats. Rate your assessment of how well you remembered something from 1 (not so good) to 5 (doing great). Make additional copies of this form to rate these techniques at different times.

RATING THE TALK ABOUT IT TECHNIQUES		
Technique Used	**Type of Information (e.g., event, book, film)**	**Rating (from 1–5)**
Just Tell It		
In reality		
Imagined interaction and speaking aloud		
Visualization and internal dialogue		
Mirror, Mirror		
In reality		
Imagined interaction and speaking aloud		
Visualization and internal dialogue		
Announcer		
In reality		
Imagined interaction and speaking aloud		
Visualization and internal dialogue		
Discuss It		
In reality		
Imagined interaction and speaking aloud		
Visualization and internal dialogue		
Teach It		
In reality		
Imagined interaction and speaking aloud		
Visualization and internal dialogue		

Share It in a Memory Group

What is a memory group? It's much like a study group, except you are not taking the same class and trying to learn the same material.

When you are seriously trying to improve your memory, as the purchase of this book suggests you are, it can be extremely helpful to find a partner or several others who are interested in doing the same. This gives you a reciprocal supply of practice partners, and a group of people with whom you can practice your memory exercises.

Any of the previous techniques are ideal for sharing in a memory group. If you have one, take turns trying out these different techniques, while others listen as an audience and interact with you.

Tell Yourself a Story

Creating stories is another way to better implant certain types of information into your memory, such as lists of items and names of people, especially when you want to remember something in a particular order. Incorporating the information into a story helps to make it more interesting and memorable, so you better encode this information in the first place. Then to retrieve it, think of the story and use the triggers within the story to retrieve the items you've planted in it. Besides helping you remember, this technique can be an enjoyable party game. It also helps to develop your imagination and can contribute to workplace bonding and motivation.

The technique is excellent to use in combination with many other techniques. For example, using visualization to create images helps you see the images as you tell the story. Or bring in other sensory modalities or anchor the story in past experiences to further reinforce and intensify the original encoding process.

The basic process is exactly what it says—you create a story that incorporates each item on a list or each name you want to remember. If the items are already in a particular order, such as a series of steps to do something, use that in organizing the story. Or to prioritize certain items, put those first in your story. Otherwise, put the list in any order. You might let the flow of the story help decide the order for you, by looking at the list and letting items pop out to come next in the story. Should more than one item come to mind as you do this, simply choose one of them to use first.

After you create the story, take a minute to focus on remembering it. Afterwards, as you remember it, write down the items or names the story refers to on your list. Notice how many names you were able to remember and compare your results to your earlier efforts to remember lists. Then, do something else for about five minutes and then use the story to recall as many words as you can. Write down those you remember and compare them to the original list. Generally, you should not only be able to remember the story but you should remember more items as you retell the story in your mind and retrieve the items in it.

When you first use this technique, start with fairly short item lists—say 7 to 12 items, since otherwise your story itself will become too long and hard to remember, defeating the whole purpose of using this method. But gradually, as your memory improves, you can increase the number of items to remember, say up to between 20 and 25 items.

You can use this technique for remembering the names of people at a party or at a business meeting, for example, or products you want to include in a presentation, or even items on a shopping list.

Creating stories can be a fun exercise and game to stimulate your imagination or enjoy yourself at a party, too. You can also use this method to make your waiting time more productive, such as looking at some objects around you and creating a story about them. (Practicing memory aids this way when the occasion arises is like exercising your brain.)

Here are some examples of how you might create a story, followed by some words you can use to create your own story. Then, try coming up with your own words by yourself or with someone else to create your stories. Finally, I've included some rules for a story-telling game that is fun for all ages; the main difference is in the particular words and the number of words you use.

Turning Words into Stories

Here are some examples of how you might create a story from some items on a list or from some names. Then, use this as a model to create your own stories.

CREATING STORIES FROM LISTS OF ITEMS OR NAMES

Items or Names on List

Shopping List:

Clock

Dress

Jeans

Paint

Cards

Hammer

Wallpaper

Ice Cream

Paper Clips

Envelopes

Story Using Items or Names on List

I woke up to the alarm **clock** ringing, so I got **dressed** quickly. I threw on a pair of **jeans.** As I ran out the door, I noticed the house needed some new **paint**, so I wrote this down on a **card**, which I **hammered** to the **wallpaper.** Then, tired from all the effort, I got some **ice cream**, and as it melted, I saw a **paper clip** on the bottom of the cup. So I put it in an **envelope** with the rest of my collection.

List of Names (using some image associations with selected names):

Barney (dinosaur)

Tom (cat)

Alice (Wonderland)

Susan (flower)

Jerry (ice cream)

Bill (dollar)

Harry (hairy ape)

Jack (cheese)

Sandy (beach)

Charlotte (spider)

When I went outside, I saw a **dinosaur** (Barney) chasing a **cat** (Tom), when suddenly **Alice** in her old-fashioned frock appeared holding a **flower** (Susan) and a big dish of **ice cream** (Jerry). Surprised, I dropped my **dollar** (Bill), and a big **hairy ape** (Harry) picked it up and ran away. But he slipped on a piece of **cheese** (Jack) on the road to the **beach** (Sandy) and was gobbled up by a huge **spider** (Charlotte).

List of Random Objects:

Elephant

River

Train

Closet

Turkey

Fish

Comb

Tree

Coffee

Car

One day an **elephant** wanted to cross the **river,** so he took a **train.** Inside, he found a big **closet.** As he looked out the window, he saw a **turkey** running by with a **fish** in his mouth and a **comb** on the top of his head. Unfortunately, he ran smack into a **tree** and fell down on a pile of **coffee** grounds. That's where a motorist in a **car** saw him and took him home for a good dinner.

Now that you have the idea, here are some lists for you to create your own story. See how fast you can do this. Try to use the words in the order they are presented, though you can change the order if it's easier for you to create a story that way.

CREATING STORIES FROM LISTS OF ITEMS OR NAMES

Items or Names on List	Story Using Items or Names on List

Shopping List:

    Camera

    Dishes

    Picture

    Towel

    Rake

    Cards

    Cake

    Lobster

    Gloves

    Hat

List of Names (using some image associations with selected names; you add the associations):

    Betty

    Dan

    Frank

    Sally

    Judy

    Miriam

    Hilda

    George

    Sam

    Henry

List of Random Objects:

    Camel

    Stairway

    Train

    Ship

    Pencil

    Snake

Notebook

Spider

Newspaper

Golf Club

After you create the story, do something else for a few minutes. Then, recall the story, and write down all the words you remember.

Now try coming up with some words and stories yourself. Build a story around the items on your real grocery list, on Saturday's chores, on the key words in your next history assignment. Start with a shorter list, say between 8 and 10 words; then as you get faster at doing this, use a longer list, say 11 to 16 words; and for an even greater challenge, come up with a list of 17 to 20 words. As you practice using this technique, your ability to both come up with stories and recall the words you are trying to remember should improve.

CREATING STORIES FROM LISTS OF ITEMS OR NAMES	
Items or Names on List	**Story Using Items or Names on List**
Shopping List:	
List of Names (using some image associations with selected names):	

Playing the Tell-Me-a-Story Game

You can use this tell-me-a-story technique to create an entertaining party game, which is a fun way to improve your memory even more.

To create the game, cut up some outline cards or heavy paper to make some small cards of about 2½ by 1½ inches. On one side of the card write down an object or name. Make about 100 of these cards. Shuffle the cards to create a deck.

Play the game with a group of three or more. In turn, a player turns up 10 cards. You can make the game harder with more cards (i.e., 11–16 cards). After receiving the cards, each player creates a story using those cards. If you want, you can turn this game into a race, where the first person to think he or she can tell a story with those words calls out "story" and tells a story. Once a player tells a story, cover up or turn over the cards.

Now everyone tries to write down as many words as they can remember in 60 seconds. If a player thinks he/she has all the words before then, he/she should call out, "Got it." When the time is up or someone calls out "Got it," everyone stops.

Turn up the words. Everyone now compares his/her words to the words on the cards. Score 1 point for correct words, minus 1 point for incorrect words, and if a person has called "Got it" and has a perfect score, he/she scores 3 extra points. Or if the person called "Got it" and made any mistakes, he/she subtracts 3 points.

While you can play multiple games with the same set of cards, create a new set with different objects and names for more variety and to avoid becoming overly familiar with the items in the deck. You'll find that not only will your memory improve as you continue to play the game, but you'll have fun.

17

Remembering a Story

While the technique in the previous chapter was focused on using stories to remember collections of words or items, the techniques in this chapter are designed to help you remember any kind of narrative, story, or sequence of events. Whether you want to tell these stories, discuss them, or write about them, these techniques can be used for:

- Telling stories to friends, associates, or others
- Remembering jokes and punch lines
- Making speeches and presentations
- Recalling topics you want to talk about in an interview
- Learning material for classes

These techniques also can be combined effectively with other techniques that increase your memory for detail, such as the use of imagery and the loci technique, discussed in Chapter 22.

The three key techniques featured here include review and rehearsal, trigger words, and word maps. These are techniques I have been using effectively myself for about three years to help me in working on additional M.A. programs, which require a lot of memory for detail.

Using Review and Rehearsal

As in remembering almost anything, review and rehearsal helps you remember by the virtue of repetition, which reinforces the information in your memory as you say it to yourself again and again. At the same time, to make your review and rehearsal more efficient, find trigger words, concepts, or summary sentences to capture the highlights. Then, as you review everything a second time, pay extra attention to these triggers, since recalling them will evoke a memory of the rest of the material in that section.

For example, here's how I've been using it to study in some English classes on mythology, children's literature, and Native American literature, where remembering the details of the story is very important. This is an approach you can adapt to learning and remembering any kind of narrative content. It is also helpful to break up the processing of new material over a period of a few days, since the consolidation that goes on in your mind overnight helps to build memory of the entire story.

First, I read over the material in full, bracketing any sections that I think are particularly important so I can read them again later. Then, the second time through, since the material is already familiar, I read it more quickly, essentially skimming for the highlights and slowing down to pay more attention to what I've already bracketed. I also use this second review as a chance to bracket any other sentences that seem especially important if I missed them the first time. In addition, I also underline one or a few key words in each paragraph, so I can use these as trigger words for each block of information.

You can use a similar approach when you are trying to remember a story, joke, or speech, so you can tell it effectively later. Review it a couple of times to get it into your long-term memory, noting any points you particularly want to mention. Then, select some trigger words for each major section of the story, and use various techniques to get these into your memory in sequence, such as the Loci Method (see Chapter 22). In a test or discussion of the material, the sequence of the story may be less important, since a question may trigger a discussion of different parts of the narrative. But when you are telling the complete story, you need a way to get those triggers in order.

Using Trigger Words

The value of trigger words is that they become a shorthand way to recall a whole section of the story or narrative. So when you go through a story or narrative you have read and underline certain words, you are selecting them to be triggers. Once you are familiar with the story through a rehearsal and review, you can focus on remembering those triggers. If you need to have them in sequence, not just recall them, use a technique for learning these words in order Then, when you think of these words in that sequence, they will call up each section of the story.

To practice this process, pick out a story or chapter in a book or an article from a magazine or newspaper. After you have read over that material, go back with a pencil or pen and highlight one or two words or phrases that seem particularly important or help to summarize the essence of that paragraph or section. After that, go back over the material again. Skim each paragraph as you do; at the same time, focus on the key words or phrases you have underlined. These will become your trigger words. Later, focus on remembering those trigger words in sequence, using any of the methods for remembering lists in sequence (such as the links system or Loci method discussed in Chapter 22.

When you create a sequence for trigger words, you can use a list or outline format. Or if you prefer, turn them into a Trigger Words Map, as described below. In this case, you lay the words out visually to help you remember.

Using a Trigger Words Map

A Trigger Words Map is a way to make the trigger words you have identified stand out graphically. It is the graphic equivalent of the Loci Method, described in Chapter 22, where you place key words or ideas in a series of locations and retrieve them as you walk the path. In this case, you create a graphic map of the key words or concepts, and you memorize that map. Afterwards, you can retrieve the key words as you make a circuit around the map. You can retrieve these words in any order, though it is helpful to retrieve the material on the branches as a group from a larger branch.

A Trigger Words Map has parallels with the idea of mind mapping used in brainstorming. However, the difference is that in a Mind Map, you put down every idea or key word for that idea that comes to mind. These maps can become extremely detailed, with dozens of words and branches. By contrast, in a Trigger Words Map, you only put down the main concepts and some key subconcepts, which trigger your memory for the rest of that idea. This way, you don't overwhelm your memory with too much of the less relevant detail, and can focus on learning the main triggers to each topic. Think of this process as putting the top two or three levels of an outline into a map format.

Here's a basic Trigger Words Map for a marketing presentation on a new health product:

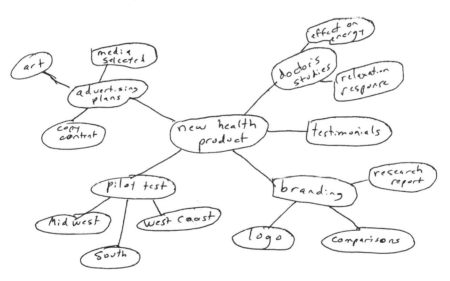

While you can just use words, you can make this Trigger Words Map more dramatic and memorable by using images or colors to highlight key points and help your recall. Or combine these words with other techniques, such as the self-referent technique, which highlights what these words and ideas mean to you.

If you use imagery, you can use your powers of visualization to associate an image with each word or concept—or only with the main concepts, while leaving the branches as just words. Or add your own simple drawings, as I have done below. Certainly, if you want to use this Trigger Words Map in a presentation, such as on a Power-Point slide, dress it up with strong imagery, say by using clip art. But if it's just for you to remember, keep it simple, as in the illustration below. You can leave the words in or not, as you prefer.

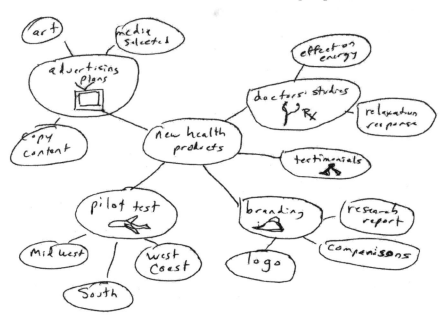

Incidentally, I'm not an artist, so in case you have trouble deciphering the images, they are the following:

- Advertising Plans = TV
- Doctors' Studies = Stethoscope and Rx Symbol
- Testimonials = Blue Ribbon Award
- Branding = Iron
- Pilot Test = Airplane

As long as you can recognize and remember the images you have drawn for yourself, that's all that matters when you are doing this just for you.

18

Back to Basics

Another type of memory aid is something you probably learned back in elementary school or high school and haven't thought of since. This basic technique is to learn new information using letters, such as acronyms and acrostics, rhymes, and jingles to remember bits of information, such as the names of the planets or the number of days in each month. How well does this method work? You probably still remember all or most of the information you memorized this way—and you may even recall it with the same trick you learned way back when.

Not only can you use already created memory aids for such basics—some of which you will find familiar—but you can create your own memory cues for whatever things you want to remember. This process works especially well for remembering up to about a dozen bits of information, such as names, places, topics to cover, or other lists of information. When you have longer material to remember, use chunking to create smaller units. You can also pull out one word to represent a longer sentence or subject you want to remember, so you can use that word for its first letter or ability to rhyme.

Here's how these different memory aids work.

Using the First Letter or Acrostics Method

In this method, you take the first letter of each word in a set you want to remember and create a word or sentence using those letters.[1]

Then, you use that word or sentence to trigger your memory for every word in the set. Hearing the first letter of each word you want to remember helps you recall the whole word. The overall category that you want to remember helps you remember, too. (For example, if you are trying to recall the colors of the rainbow, each word will be a color.) Here are some popular memory cues that have been used:

- ROY G. BIV (the colors of the rainbow—red, orange, yellow, green, blue, indigo, violet).

- Every good boy does fine (the musical notes on the lines of a treble cleft: EGBDF).²

- Green bananas help sister nations create prosperity (the countries of Central America, in order from North America to South America—Guatemala, Belize, Honduras, El Salvador, Nicaragua, Costa Rica, Panama).

- My very educated mother just sliced up nine pickles (the order of the planets in the solar system—Mercury, Venus, Earth, Mars, Jupiter, Saturn, Uranus, Neptune, Pluto—although now there will need to be a new memory cue, since Pluto just got demoted and is no longer a planet!)

- Phyllis came over for Gene's special variety (the categories for classifying plants and animals in biology, which I learned in elementary school—Phylum, Class, Order, Genus, Species, Variety).

Similarly, you can use this approach to help you remember a grocery list, names of people in a group, tasks to complete each day, and so forth. Here's an example to get you started; practice creating some of your own lists using the chart below. Then, turn the first letter of each item on the list into a word or the first word of a sentence.

FIRST LETTER WORDS OR SENTENCES TO REMEMBER	
Items to Remember	Acrostic to Use
Grocery List for Party: Peanuts, Almonds, Bread, Chocolate, Milk, Cake, Fudge, Apples, Pie	Phil and Brad chose more candy for a party.

Using Acronyms

Acronyms are much like acrostics in that they use the first letter of each word in a set or series to create another word or easy to remember combination of letters. But the difference between acrostics and acronyms is that in acronyms, the letters combine to form a single word or collection of letters. And sometimes an acronym uses a second letter from a word in the series, most commonly a vowel, to make the acronym easier to read.[3] And often a small word like "of" or "and" is dropped in creating the acronym.

You will be familiar with many of the acronyms that are in common use, such as the FBI for the Federal Bureau of Investigation (an example of dropping the "of") and NASA for the National Aeronautics and Space Administration (an example of dropping the "and"). In fact, many times the names of organizations, particularly in the government, are shortened to acronyms, and some common terms in science and technology actually started off as acronyms. For example, "radar" is an acronym for radio detecting and ranging (and an example of taking two letters from a word for easier reading). Even if an organization doesn't have a common acronym or you don't know it on hearing the full name, you can easily create one yourself, such as the Bureau of Homeland Security (BHS).

You may also be familiar with some acronyms used to help you remember items in school, such as HOMES, used for the five great lakes—Huron, Ontario, Michigan, Erie, and Superior.

You can also create your own acronym to help you remember a short list of items or tasks to do—up to about six or seven.

Here's an example to get you started. Then practice creating some acronyms yourself using the chart below. Just take the first letter of each item on the list to create an acronym (and use the rule about taking the first two letters or dropping small words to make the word as appropriate).

USING ACRONYMS TO REMEMBER	
Items to Remember	**Acronym to Use**
Tasks to Do for Presentation: Prepare handouts. Take business cards. Take PowerPoint CD. Take airline printout. Pack suitcases.	HB-PAP

Using Rhymes and Jingles

Rhymes and jingles are still another way to learn and remember new material. A jingle is basically a rhyme set to music so you can sing it.

You have probably learned a number of these in elementary, junior high, and high school to help you remember new concepts and historical references; they are a common device on TV programs for preschool children, such as *Sesame Street*. Using a verse or a catchy tune helps to make the topic more exciting and fun, and therefore more memorable.

For example, some of the rhymes and jingles I remember from school—yes, even after not thinking about them for decades—include these:

- For remembering the dates of the month:

  Thirty days has September,
  April, June, and November.
  All the rest have thirty-one
  Except for February,
  Which has twenty-eight or twenty-nine.

- For remembering when Columbus discovered America:

  Columbus sailed the ocean blue
  In 1492.

- For learning spelling:

  I before *e*
  Except after *c*.

Rhymes and jingles are often used in advertising to make an ad more memorable, such as this rhyme that I remember from childhood. (In fact, I won a contest to make up other ad jingles for the product—though ironically, I can't remember my own submission.)

You'll wonder where the yellow went
When you brush your teeth with Pepsodent.

Think about what rhymes and jingles you have used in the past, and if you feel creatively inspired, create your own rhymes and jingles to help you remember something. Here's an example of how you might create your own rhyme or jingle. Then, try creating your own for tasks you have to do. (Or create these with your family members as a fun way to help them remember to do certain tasks.)

USING RHYMES AND JINGLES TO REMEMBER	
Items to Remember	**Rhyme or Jingle to Use**
Things to Get at the Store:	
Jacket	I need a jacket and a coat.
Coat	Have to get some shoes and socks.
Shoes	And don't forget to go
Socks	To the drugstore for a clock.
Clock	
Tasks to Do at Home:	
Take out garbage.	Pick up the trash.
Clean up kitchen.	And do the dishes.
Get the laundry on the way home.	Get the laundry.
Get fish food.	And feed the fishes.

These basic ways of making things memorable can also be a fun way to get friends, family, or work group members to remember to do something. For example, in *The Great Memory Book*, Karen Markowitz and Eric Jensen describe how rhymes were used to teach children the household rules in a fun way, such as: "When you're sick, you get your pick. . . . When you're tall enough to touch your toes, you're big enough to pick up your clothes. . . . Take what you're served, eat what you wish, and leave the rest upon your dish."[4]

19

Take a Letter

Just as there are a number of memory strategies that use numbers (see Chapter 28), so there are different strategies based on letters. You have to first select the letters and associated images, and learn them well. After that, you can use them to help you remember combinations of letters, such as a password—or combine them with one of the number systems when you have a string of letters and numbers. This is a system I don't use, since I prefer chunking, rehearsal, and keeping everything in a file of passwords, but many memory experts swear by these kinds of systems—so here goes.

The Alphabet System

To start, pick a word with a visual image associated with it (such as "apple") that starts with each letter or with the sound of the letter in the alphabet. It's probably good to pick a different image than you are using to remember a number, so you don't get them confused. Should a letter make a word, such as where the letter "J" forms the word "jay" or "B" forms the word "bee," use that word. You can also use initials that create a meaningful word, such as "U.N." for the letter "U."

Memory expert Tony Buzan recommends choosing a word that begins with the sound of the letter, such as "elephant" for the letter "L"[1] or "eye" for the letter "I." But if I were using the system, I

181

would prefer to use words that actually start with that letter, even though they don't have the same sound, such as "lock" for "L" or "brick" for "B."

Conversely, Buzan recommends not using words that don't start with the sound of the letter as you pronounce it when you say the alphabet, such as the words "ant" for "A," "bottle" for "B," "dog" for "D," and "eddy" for "E." Again, I wouldn't do it this way. Perhaps the difference is that I have a strong visual imagery, so I see the letters associated with the word in my mind's eye, so it feels more natural to use a word that begins with the letter. By contrast, if I used a sound-alike word with a different letter, like "elephant" for the letter "L," the first thing that would come to mind for me is the letter "E." Use whatever approach feels right for you—choosing an alphabet word with that same letter or that same sound, although sometimes—and ideally—a word will be both, providing both visual and aural reinforcement.

Choosing Your Words

Following are letters with some possible words you can use, based on using both the visual and sound-alike systems. I have listed the same word when it both starts with the same letter and sounds alike. Use one of those—or choose your own word.

ALPHABET WORD IMAGES			
Letter	Visual Image	Sound-Alike Image	Your Image Choice
A	Ace	Ace	
B	Bee	Bee	
C	Cake	Sea	
D	Deed, Duck	Deed, DDT	
E	Easel	Easel	
F	Farm	Effervescence	
G	Garage	Jeep, Jeans	

H	Hanger	H-bomb	
I	Ice	Eye	
J	Jay	Jay	
K	Kangaroo	Cake	
L	Lamp	Elastic, Elbow	
M	Milk	MC (emcee)	
N	Nail	Entire, Energy	
O	Oboe	Oboe	
P	Pea	Pea	
Q	Queue	Queue	
R	Rack	Arch	
S	Snake	Eskimo	
T	Tea, T-Square	Tea, T-Square	
U	Umbrella	Yew, Ewe	
V	Vehicle, V.P.	Vehicle, V.P.	
W	Wagon	W.C.	
X	X-Ray	X-Ray	
Y	Yurt	Wife	
Z	Zebra	Zebra	

Building Image Associations

Okay, now that you have chosen your word, visualize an image of that word in your mind and draw that image to help reinforce that association. You can use the following chart to draw this.

ALPHABET WORD DRAWINGS: A–Z		
Letter	**Image**	**Drawing of Image**
A		
B		
C		
D		
E		
F		
G		
H		
I		
J		
K		
L		
M		
N		
O		
P		
Q		
R		
S		
T		
U		

V		
W		
X		
Y		
Z		

Now practice learning these associations, just as you would learn the associations with numbers and images. First, visualize the image in your mind, as you go down the list, letter by letter. Then, reverse the order and try to recall the image. Finally, think of the letters in a random order and try to remember them.

Lastly, practice with a few combinations of letters, coming up with stories or incidents that link the images together. Start with four or five letters; then expand the number of letters you do this for. Finally, try doing this for combinations of letters and numbers, which are often combined together in a password.

For example, say the letters you are trying to remember are JXTB—You might imagine a blue *jay* flying into an *x-ray* machine and falling into a glass of *tea,* after which he is stung by a *bee.* Use whatever image words you have come up with in creating these stories, whether you prefer look-alike or sound-alike words to help you remember.

Playing the Learn Your Letters Game

As in the case of numbers, you might find it fun to play a letter game. For example, if you come across some letters while you are waiting on a ticket line or for the bus or subway, come up with a story using your associations with that number.

Or you may want to create a game to practice with others learning the system, where you race to come up with stories when you see a series of letters or a word. Or seek to create the most interesting and unique story. Alternatively, take turns picking out a series of letters, say from a Scrabble game, and tell a story with the images associated with those letters. Then, the other players race to be the first to come up with the correct letter combination or word. Win a point for being the first; lose a point if you are incorrect in stating the letter series or word. The player with the most points when the game ends wins.

20

Linked In and Linked Up

Linking up is a powerful way of making connections so you can remember short lists. This system is a very basic introduction to using your imagination to create links—even more basic than creating a story. Think of it as a way to incorporate a variety of memory principles and limber up your memory muscle, so you can apply these methods for even more elaborate systems. Linking is most appropriate for remembering short lists, from grocery lists to the subjects you want to cover in a meeting or speech.

Essentially, you help make your memories more memorable by using your mind proactively to make your memories more vivid through imagery and associations. Then, you either create a continuous narrative that links all of the images together in sequence, or you link a series of pairs of items like a chain, where you create a visual association between the first two items, then between the second and third item, the third and fourth, and so on. I call these the "continuous link system" and the "chain link system." In either case, you use various memory-sharpening skills that increase recall. You might even close your eyes to cut out distractions, hone your concentration, and make the imagery more vivid when you first are learning to visualize, though as you become accustomed to creating images in your mind's eye, you can do this anywhere, anytime.

According to memory expert Tony Buzan in his book *Use Your*

Perfect Memory, the sharpening skills that improve memory include the following (which I have described in a little more detail):

- *Using the Five Senses—Sight, Hearing, Touch, Smell, and Taste,* where the more fully you experience something, in reality or in your mind, the more it will come to mind in the future.

- *Movement:* where you incorporate motion in your visualization—or move yourself.

- *Association:* whereby you associate one thing with another to trigger a memory when you see or experience the association.

- *Sexuality:* where a sexual association creates a stimulus that is more exciting and therefore more memorable.

- *Humor:* where the experience of laughter and amusement makes the memory more pleasurable, and hence something you more want to remember.

- *Imagination:* where you use your creativity to add oomph to your desired memory.

- *Number:* where you group things together, as in chunking, to make memory easier.

- *Symbolism:* where you associate things you want to remember with symbols that help you remember.

- *Color:* where you make any imagery more vivid and hence more memorable.

- *Order and Sequence:* where you arrange things into an order based on common characteristics, priority, numerical sequence, or other organizing principles.

- *Positive Images:* where you emphasize the positive, because you arc more apt to remember what's pleasurable (as we learned earlier, we repress negative experiences because we don't want to think about them).

- *Exaggeration:* where you make things even bigger and grander than they are, so they stand out in your memory.

- *Absurdity:* where you make something very crazy, bizarre, and outlandish to help it stand out in your mind.

- *Substitution:* where you replace something you want to remember with something else you can remember even better, and then, through the power of association you recall what the substitution represents.

The reason these principles work, according to memory experts, is that you use both sides of your brain—both your left and right cortex. So you not only use a more analytical approach to remembering associated with your left cortex (such as chunking and rehearsing), but you tap into your more intuitive and holistic side with your right cortex as you create visual and sensual images. It's like the difference between putting something you want to remember in a beautifully framed picture that stands out in your mind or into a file in a musty file cabinet that you have to burrow through to find that document again.

Using the Continuous Link System

In the continuous link system, you create a narrative link for each item on the list in sequence.

To practice with this system, take any short list of things you want to remember, even very mundane items on a shopping list, create a series of associations for each item, and link those together into a sequence as you travel through time or space. For example, imagine you are taking a walk or driving in a car, and as you go along, you see each item. But more than that, use other principles of memory, such as exaggeration and absurdity, to make these images even more memorable. Some of the possible trips you might take as you make these link-ups include a walk in the park, a flower garden, or your neighborhood, or a drive through the country.

Then, as you go on this journey, you see the items you want to remember.

For example, here's how you might apply the various memory principles with the following everyday shopping list: apples, eggs, soap, sugar, coffee, ice cream, paper cups, pie, bread, and fish.

Say you are going for a walk in the country. First you pass an apple tree, but these are not ordinary apples. You **see** they are **col-**

ored with all the hues of the rainbow, and you suddenly **hear** them start **singing**.

As you look down, you **see** some very **large** eggs, the size of footballs, and you reach down and **touch** them. When you do, they start **moving**, by rolling around and bouncing up and down.

As they do this, you discover they are bouncing on a large, white bar of soap, which is shaped like a boat, so you start **laughing** because you think it's so funny. Then, as it floats off, you see nearby a lake made of white sugar, a truly **absurd** picture, and next to it you **hear** the sound of a bubbling brook, and it is the **color** of coffee. But is it? You reach down to dip your finger in the brook, and as you **touch** it, you **smell** the sweet coffee, which makes you hungry. So you reach out and grab a big, round ball of ice cream that is hanging from the trees like a ball of fruit.

As you pull each ball off the tree, you put it in a **huge**, spinning paper cup in front of you. Then, to test your aim, you step away, and pick up some pies and **throw** them at the cup, so you will win a reward—a **great, big** teddy bear made of bread. And after you make several successful throws you get the first prize—a **gigantic** fish that you can frame to show what a great catch you made.

In short, you have made a series of associations that link the items on your list together, using the many principles that help to make a powerful memory.

Okay, now that you understand the basic principles through reading the fantasy, without looking back at the original list or the fantasy, see how many items you can remember. You can use that number as a baseline when you try your own lists, create your own linked associations using these principles, and then try to remember even longer lists.

HOW MUCH CAN YOU REMEMBER? (Write down as many items as you can from the shopping list.)	

Now, start creating your own lists. These can be random lists of anything, or pick out some items on a list you really want to remember.

Once you have selected your items, create your own fantasies using the above memory principles, making them as vivid and creative as possible. Afterwards, test yourself again and see how many items on your list you remembered. Additionally, check how many you remembered in the proper order. In some cases, just remembering the items is sufficient, but sometimes, such as when you are giving a speech, you want to remember the precise order, so you link different sections of it to a path through your house.

You can also turn this process into a game you play with others, which makes improving your memory even more fun—and memorable. Here's how.

Playing the Linking Game

Decide how many items you want to remember (7 is a good starting point, but you can work your way up to 10 or more pretty quickly). Then, each person creates a list on a card on a sheet of paper or index card. Now mix up the lists and give each person a list other than their own.

Each person will now read his/her list aloud in turn, allowing about 10 seconds between items, so each person can create their own fantasy associations with that image. After the person has read his/

her complete list, everyone else will write down as many items on the list as they can remember in the next minute or two.

When everyone has finished, read the list aloud again, and each person other than the person reading the list gets 2 points for each item correctly remembered in the correct order, 1 point for each item remembered but out of order, and loses 1 point for each item that doesn't belong on the list.

Go around the group so everyone has a chance to be the reader. At the end, total the scores for each round, and the person with the highest score wins.

As a variation in play, after the reader reads the whole list and players write down the words they can remember, each person in turn relates his or her fantasy for those words—which can help everyone in developing their imagination. You might even vote on who has created the most imaginative story, with the winner for each round being the person who has gotten the most votes. The overall winner is the person who has won the most rounds.

Using the Chain Link System

In the chain link system, as described by numerous memory experts, including Kenneth L. Higbee in his book *Your Memory: How It Work & How to Improve It,* you create a series of short image associations that link each item in the list to the previous item, rather than crafting a continuous narrative. This system is also ideal for remembering all of the items in order.

The way the process works is you create a visual image for each item in the list and then you associate the image for one item with the next item on the list. We can use the same list as above: apples, eggs, soap, sugar, coffee, ice cream, paper cups, pie, bread, and fish.

You might create the following chain link of associations, incorporating the principles described above to make the imagery dramatic and memorable.

To associate **apples** and **eggs,** imagine the apples falling from a tree in an orchard and landing on top of a line of eggs, with a big SPLAT!

To associate **eggs** and **soap**, imagine someone throwing eggs at some bars of soap, which are targets in a competition.

To associate **soap** and **sugar,** imagine a small boy using a bar of soap in a bathtub, when he sees a big monster made of **sugar.**

To associate **sugar** with **coffee,** imagine the big sugar monster striding forward through a river of brown coffee.

And so on. The imagery for each association doesn't have to carry over from each paired link in the chain, although it can, such as in the case of the image of the sugar monster in both paired associations.

Have fun making these associations. You also can play the same game described above with the chained links, instead of using continuous links.

21

Find a Substitute

If you can't make a meeting or event, you often may be able to get help by having a stand-in attend for you. Sometimes the substitute can even do it better than you.

Well, the same principle works in memory. If you have trouble learning or remembering a difficult word or name, especially a foreign one, you can better remember if you use a sub. This technique is ideal for remembering either unfamiliar words in English or foreign words.

Using the Sub System to Remember Single Words

Again, you use the principle of imagery and associations to create a connection between the word you want to remember and visualizations that make the word more memorable. As Harry Lorayne and Jerry Lucas describe in *The Memory Book*, "When you hear or see a word or phrase that seems abstract or intangible to you, think of something—anything—that sounds like, or reminds you of, the abstract material and *can be pictured in your mind.*"[1]

For example, the state name of Minnesota would become "mini soda," a small bottle of soda, while Mississippi might become "Mrs. Sip." Then, if you want to remember these in order, use the continuous or chain link system to create an association, such as a mini soda in a very small bottle and a married woman sipping from the small bottle.[2]

Or say you want to learn a new word like "endocarp"—which means a fruit pit. You might imagine yourself "ending" the carp by imagining yourself hitting the fish, with a very large fruit pit—an association suggested by Harry Lorayne in his *Page-A-Minute Memory Book*.[3]

Likewise, if you are struggling to learn foreign words, you can apply the same principle. For instance, as suggested by Lorayne,[4] to remember the French word for father, *père*, you might think of a large pear holding a baby in its arms, so you associate the substitute word with the meaning of the French word for father.

To remember the Japanese word *sayonara*, which means goodbye, you might see yourself sighing on air as you bid your goodbyes.

This same principle applies to remembering the long and often convoluted names of drugs or unusual food dishes. For example, take the hard-to-remember word *hydrochlorothiazine,* which is a medicine to take for high blood pressure. (Hopefully you won't be needing it as you try to learn the principles in the book.) You might think of these associations:

- Hydro—a plane with skis for landing on the water or a water plant
- Chloro—a rainbow of colors with a big "HL" sign in the middle of it
- Thi—a shapely woman's thigh
- Zine—a magazine on a Website, which is in fact called a "zine"

Or say you are trying to remember the name of the French vegetable stew *ratatouille*. You might think of a "rat" on a hotel roof climbing on a big letter "A," falling down on a large number "2" on a hotel sign, and being chased by a "wee" little man.

The same principle can apply to remembering unusual names of people—or any names for that matter. For example, you are introduced to a man named Anthony Coddington. For the first name "Anthony," you might think of an "aunt" and "honey," visualizing your favorite aunt collecting honey from a hive. For the last name "Coddington," you might visualize a "cod," a ringing phone for "ding," and a heavy weight with the writing "1 ton" on it. In short, you use compelling images to substitute for the syllables in the name, and then when you see that person again, the pictures you have created lead you to quickly recall the person's name.

Using Substitutes to Create Links

Besides using the substitution system to remember single words, you can use additional associations, such as between the word and its meaning, a state name and its capital, a name and a face, a person to an address, company, or phone number, and so on.

For example, to use another example adapted from Lorayne's *Memory Book*, to remember that the capital city of Maryland is Annapolis, think of a beautiful girl named **Mary land**ing on **an apple.**

Or supposed you want to remember that your new acquaintance Anthony Coddington is the CEO of the Redstone Mills Company. Use the imagery associated with his name above (your **aunt** collecting **honey** from a hive, a **cod**fish lying beside a phone with a **ding** sound, and a 1 **ton** weight), and then see your aunt picking up a large **red stone** and taking it to a **mill.**

Practicing the Sub System

Now that you've gotten the basic idea, start practicing to put the sub system into operation.

Come up with your own list, such as by looking in a dictionary, foreign language book, phone book, or ad for drugs. Pick words you are interested in learning and are having trouble with. Say you are taking a class in a foreign language, are learning the names of families and species in a birding or biology class, or are trying to learn specialized words in a professional discipline. Each of these situations would involve unfamiliar words that you might need to learn.

First, break each word down into a series of substitute image words. Then, take some time to visualize the image associations to form the memory link.

Playing the Sub Words Game

To enhance your ability to use this technique, as well as have fun with it, play the Sub Words game with a group of people.

You can play it in two ways:

1. *Sub Words Charades.* Play individually—or if you have enough people, divide into pairs. In turn, each person or team will come up with a long word, foreign word, or personal name; secretly divide it into a series of images suggesting the whole word or a syllable of it, and indicate what category the substitute word is in. Then, as you take turns acting out those images, others will call out what the image is. The first person to get the image right gets a point. Keep going until all the images are identified or someone gets the whole correct word or name and scores an additional 3 points for that.

   The winner is the player or team with the highest score after a complete round or series of rounds in which all players come up with and act out a word for the round.

2. *Sub Words Picture Race.* As in Sub Words Charades, you can play individually or form into pairs. Similarly, come up with a word or name and a series of images for each word or syllable, and say how many syllables it is. The difference here is that instead of acting out the images for the word, draw a picture of it, and show it to the group. The person who calls out the full word or name correctly scores 5 points. But otherwise, no one scores.

   Then, show a second image picture besides the first. Again, anyone can call out the full word or name correctly and scores 5 points if they do.

   But be careful in calling out your guesses that you don't make a near miss and give away the correct answer to someone else.

   The person with the highest score wins.

It's All About Location

One of the oldest memory aids is the method of "loci," or locations—sometimes called the "journey technique." According to memory experts, this technique dates back at least to the Greek orators, who used this approach to remember their compelling speeches. Supposedly, Simonides of Ceos, born in the 6th century B.C., was the first to develop memory training, and he created the "loci technique" of mentally placing bits of information at different locations so the orators would find it easier to remember them.[1] These orators may have also called on the help of the Greek goddess of memory, Mnemosyne, the source of the word *mnemonic*.[2] The Romans further adapted this system into the Roman Room system.

But the significance of place in memories can go back much further. One can even imagine preliterate storytellers, with their long-standing oral tradition, using such a method to remember their long stories about gods, animals, ancestors, and how things came to be. In fact, they often connected stories to all aspects of nature—from stories about the sun, moon, and stars to nearby trees, plants, rocks, and animals.

Using the Loci Method

Using the Loci Method is a little like that, because you are imagining different words, objects, or ideas associated with different locations.

They could be places from your favorite walk in the park, from a walk around your house or office, or any location you choose.

The method is especially useful when you want to learn a series of items—from words and names to topics to cover in a speech—in a particular order. Commonly, the method is used to go from place to place in a particular order. But as you get better at using this method, there's no reason why you can't zero in on a particular location to trigger your memory for what's there—or even go backwards on the route in reverse order.

The method is also ideally suited to be used for a location you already know well, such as your home or office. As you walk through the location, you pick out places that you want to associate with a particular item. For instance, in your home, you might start by pulling your car in the **driveway,** then go along the **path** to your **front door,** open that and step into the **hallway,** after which you go into the **living room, kitchen,** and **den** and go up the stairs to the **master bedroom,** a smaller **bedroom,** and finally to the **hall closet.** You can select these places either in your imagination or by actually taking a walk to see them. Just pick out places that form a logical path as you walk around from start to finish.

If you are using your office, some stops along the way might be the building **lobby,** the **elevator** to your floor, the **hallway** outside your office, the **reception desk,** the **corridor** from the reception area to the offices, the **kitchen** or **snack area,** your **boss's office, your own office,** and a **co-worker's office.** Likewise, if you are into nature walks, pick out distinctive spots along a trail you know well. Or pick out a series of stops on a walk around a local park or city street.

Then, to associate a particular word, item, topic, concept, or idea with each location, make up an image to represent it; finally, individually associate each word, item, topic, concept, or idea with that location. Make the image visually exciting to help you better remember the image. The more dramatic, even bizarre and wacky the scene, the better you can remember it.[3]

After you come up with the associations, write them down to help affix them in your memory. After that, you can go back and review your associations with these items and locations to help implant them in your memory.

Here's an example of how you might use the Loci Method to remember a grocery list using your home. Say your grocery list includes 10 items: hamburgers, dog food, apples, bananas, orange juice, ice cream, tomato soup, milk, soap, and plastic wrap. You might turn this into a series of associations such as this:

- As you pull your car in the **driveway** you see a man jumping up and down eating a **hamburger**.
- When you go along the **path,** you see a big dog coming to lick your face, because he is hungry for some **dog food**.
- At your **front door,** you see a long snake hanging from the top of the door with a big **apple** in his mouth.
- In the **hallway,** you see two children fencing with **bananas**.
- When you walk into the **living room,** you see painters with buckets of **orange juice** who are painting the room orange.
- In the **kitchen,** you see a huge snowman made of vanilla **ice cream** instead of snow.
- In the **den** you see a body lying under the desk, like in a Hollywood film, and you see that he has **tomato soup** on his shirt in place of blood.
- In the **master bedroom,** you encounter a beautiful nymph who is sitting in a bathtub of **milk**.
- In a smaller **bedroom,** you see a big bar of **soap** that suddenly expands and expands and turns into a cloud of soap bubbles.
- Finally, in the **hall closet,** you discover a mummy enclosed in **plastic wrap**.

So now that you've got the idea, here's a list of places in the office and a list of things to take with you to a meeting. See what kinds of images you can come up with for them:

- The building **lobby—briefcase**
- The **elevator** to your floor—**PowerPoint presentation**

- The **hallway** outside your office—**projector**
- The **reception desk—notebook**
- The **corridor** from the reception area to the offices—**camera**
- The **kitchen** or **snack area—coat**
- Your **boss's office—screen**
- **Your own office—note cards**
- A **coworker's office—books**

Similarly, you can use this method to cover different topics, such as when you have to come up with trigger words for outlining or mapping out a talk or for listing the things you need to remember for a test on a subject.

You can increase or decrease the number of stops along the way depending on your number of items. However, if the number of locations becomes too great, you may have trouble remembering all of them. If so, try combining two or three items together at one location. For example, in the shopping list example, you might put the **hamburger, dog food,** and **apple** in the **driveway**, and imagine a scene that connects all three items, such as: As you come into the driveway, you see the man who is jumping up and down eating a **hamburger** suddenly get down on all fours, turn into a dog, and start eating **dog food** out of a bowl. Then, a little kid from next door rolls an **apple** at the bowl, knocking it over, whereupon the dog starts barking.

You can use the same location more than once if there is a time lapse between the different items you want to remember, particularly if you are going to use a set of completely different items. With a sufficient time delay, your memory from one list generally won't proactively interfere with your memory of the next set of items. But otherwise, it might be better to use a different setting for a different list to reduce the chances of mixing up different items associated with the same location.

Researchers have found that this technique can be effective even when there is a delay in calling up the items associated with each location. For example, Margaret Matlin reports that in one classic experiment, participants who used the Loci Method to remember a list of words were able to remember about twice as many words five weeks later as others who were simply told to remember the words.[4]

Working with the Loci Method

The chart below will help you practice using these methods. You can walk through the location in reality or in your mind. Use as many locations as you have items, but if you have more than 12 or 16 items, put 2 or more items at each location. Write down each stop on the journey, then write down a brief reference to the association you are making.

LOCATION		
Location	Item to Remember	Association

Using the Roman Room System

While the Loci or Journey Method is based on going on a journey through a familiar place, the "Roman Room" system involves creating a room in a house in your imagination; then you fill it with any pieces of furniture or objects that you want. But keep the room orderly, so you can more easily move around it to mentally move from object to object. Thereafter, those items become the link to which you attach an image of what you want to remember. As in the loci method, create as dramatic an image as possible for this.

In *Use Your Perfect Memory*, Tony Buzan, an expert on brain and learning techniques, gives an example for how a Roman might have used this method. In his imagination, the Roman might have envisioned a room with two large pillars at the front door, a carved lion's head on the doorknob, and a Greek statue in the hallway. Next to the statue, he might have imagined a flowering plant.[5]

Then, as Buzan describes, the Roman might have imagined an ancient Roman version of a to-do list in this way.[6] Say his to-do list included buying a pair of sandals, getting his sword sharpened, finding a new servant, taking care of his grapevine, and polishing his helmet. He might begin the memory process this way:

- At the first stop, the left-hand pillar, he would imagine hundreds of hanging sandals, and not only see the glistening leather but smell it and touch it.

- At the second stop, the right-hand pillar, he would see himself sharpening his sword, and additionally experience the sound of the scraping and feel the blade becoming sharper and sharper.

- At the third stop, the carved lion's head doorknob, he would imagine the servant he plans to buy riding the lion.

- At the fourth stop, the Greek statue, he would imagine the grapes of his grapevine encircling the statue, and he might not only see the grapes but experience tasting them.

- And at the fifth stop, the flowering plant next to the statue, he might see his helmet hanging from a flower.

Well, you get the idea. You use your imagination to create a lot of vivid and sensual images—and the room itself is entirely imaginary, unlike the familiar location you use in the Loci Method, so you can let your imagination run wild. As Buzon describes it:

> The delight of this system is that the room is *entirely* imaginary, so you can have in it every wonderful item that you wish; things that please all your senses, items of furniture and objects of art you have always desired to possess in real life, and similarly foods and decorations that especially appeal to you . . .
>
> The Roman Room system eliminates all boundaries on your imagination and allows you to remember as many items as you wish.[7]

In fact, Buzon suggests that when you use this system, as you imagine yourself possessing certain objects in your imaginary room, both your memory and your creative intelligence will work subconsciously so you may eventually acquire those objects[8]—such as if you envision a car you always wanted in the center of the room.

You can use the following chart to write down the items you would like to have in your memory room; then draw your room with these objects in it. Put as many objects in the room as you like—though initially you might start with about 7 to 10 objects; later you can always add more objects.

As the number of items in your memory room expands, you can write these down and draw your room on a larger sheet of paper.

Once you have selected the items for your room and drawn them on a sheet of paper, take a walk around your room several times in your memory. As you do, carefully encode into your memory the exact order and position of all the items in your room. Use all of your senses as you do this, so you not only visualize what's there, but listen to what's in the room, smell any smells, touch the items, and taste anything that's there to taste, like the luscious box of candy on the brown oak table by the sofa with green velvet cushions. This process will help to implant this room in your memory.

Then, with this room clearly in mind, place objects you want to

ITEMS FOR MY MEMORY ROOM

Furniture and Other Objects I Want in My Memory Room

My Memory Room

remember along the path you take through your room and create vivid associations.

Again, you can use a single image for each object in the room—or as the number of items to remember expands, place two or three items at each location. Also, allow a little time to go by before you use this room to remember another list of items, so you don't get the associations confused. Or, create a second Roman Room to remember different items.

Applying the Loci and Roman Room Methods

As previously noted, these methods are ideal when you want to re-member lists of anything—from shopping lists to to-do lists to topics in a speech. But what if you have several lists to remember? How often can you use the same location?

One way to apply these methods is to vary which method you use for different lists to reduce the chances that you will have imag-ery from a past list intruding on a new one. For instance, use the Loci Method for a shopping list and use the Roman Room method for a list of topics to cover in a presentation.

Generally, after a few days, you can use a familiar location or the room for remembering another set of information. Or if you have multiple lists of items to remember in one day, you might use a dif-ferent location or create another room to use for additional lists of items.

Find out what works for you. If you don't get any proactive inter-ference from a past list when you memorize your new lists, it's fine to keep using the same location or room. But if you do have interfer-ence, change locations and rooms so you make new associations be-tween them and the items you want to remember.

Additionally, you might choose a location or room that is partic-ularly applicable to the information you want to remember. For ex-ample, if you want to remember a personal to-do list, use the living room; for the names of clients at work, use your office; for the names of hit songs and movies, use a recreation room; and so on. Fit the location to what you want to remember and that'll help you remem-ber better, through even stronger associations, because of the power of context.

Finally, you must practice to firmly fix the locations or places in the room in your imagination, so you can easily walk through each place and remember what is there in order. Once the stops on the journey are firmly fixed in your imagination, you can easily locate items out of order. You just see the place, call up your association with it, and you will remember the item on your list that you have placed there.

23

Be a Recorder

Another powerful way to remember what you observe or experience is to imagine yourself as a camera or audio recorder. The purpose of these techniques is to remind you to pay extra attention to details, so you pick up and record even more. Then, you have more complete and firmly encoded material for better recall later.

The basic way these techniques work is that you use a trigger you have created, such as snapping your fingers a certain way or telling yourself that "Now I am a camera . . . Now I am a tape recorder." Then, you go into record mode, where you pay extra careful attention to whatever you are observing, hearing, or otherwise experiencing. By reminding yourself to use either of these techniques, you are more alert and attentive, so you take in more detailed information. Chapter 5 introduced some exercises to help you enhance your powers of observation.

Pick out the times when you want to use one of these techniques, since it might be too tiring to stay continually at this heightened state of alert. You might find you are overwhelmed by information overload. But used selectively, being a camera or audio recorder can truly enhance how much you can remember. For example, I used these techniques when I was doing participant observation research for sociology and anthropology. I couldn't take notes or use a tape recorder, since this would unnerve the people who were in the study, so I had to remember as much as I could as accurately and in as much detail as possible. Typically, these periods of intense observation and listening went on for about one to three hours, though sometimes they lasted all day. As soon as I got home, I would go to my typewriter or computer (yes, I did once use a typewriter when I first started doing this research in the mid-1970s), and write up my notes—what sociologists and anthropologists call "field notes." Thinking of myself as a video camera or tape recorder helped me to experience what was happening more intensely in the first place, so I was able to recall more later.

When you use these techniques, it's best to recall what you can soon after the experience you recorded. Otherwise, as you start to do other things, the memory will fade and you won't be able to get as much detail.

Now here's a more detailed description of each technique. Try putting them into practice in different situations. Then, within an hour or two, see how much detail you can remember as you write down your notes on what you experienced. As you continue to practice these techniques, your ability to both encode and retrieve more detail will improve. At the end of this chapter are tips to help you keep track of your progress in using these techniques.

I Am a Camera

In the "I am a camera" technique, imagine that you are either a still camera or video camera. As you look, imagine there are frames around whatever you are looking at, and observe closely.

I am a Still Camera

With a still camera, you can really zero in on the scene, so this is an especially good technique for something that has little motion, such as looking at scenery, a room in a house, or a picture in an art gallery or museum. Imagine you are taking a photograph of the scene and carefully observe everything in the picture. Notice the colors, shapes, lines, objects, people, and the relationship of one object or person to another. You can look at the overall scene or zoom in to focus on an area of the photo you find especially interesting.

In practicing with this technique, take a minute or two to carefully observe. A minute is fine if this is a relatively simple shot, but if there's lots of detail, take two minutes. Test yourself by either writing down everything you observed in the photo or drawing what you observed. Afterwards, look back at the scene and score 1 point for everything you recognized and subtract 1 point for everything you incorrectly put in the picture, to get your score. Last, count up the number of different objects or people in the scene and divide your score by the total to get your rating as a percentage. You should find as you continue to use this technique that your score will increase over time.

I am a Video Camera

Instead of seeing what you are observing as a still camera, you see everything in motion. To start the process, imagine a frame around what you are looking at, and imagine that you are filming with a video camera. Imagine that you are either the camera or the person looking through the lens.

Then, pay careful attention to what you see on the screen. As with the still camera technique, notice the colors, shapes, lines, objects, people, and relationship of one object or person to another. You can look at the overall scene or zoom in to focus on an area of the screen you find especially interesting. In addition, notice any movement or interaction between the people in the scene. If you are close enough, include audio, and listen closely to what people are saying; otherwise, just focus on what you observe.

The technique is best suited to anything that involves movement, from making observations from your own moving vehicle to observing a meeting or interaction between two people or going to a sporting event. Later, imagine that you hit the replay button and replay the scene in your mind. As you replay the scene, carefully look at what you see. To focus in on specific details, hit your mental pause button, and look more closely. Release it to continue the scene.

You can't test yourself as precisely with the video camera technique as with the still camera technique, since everything is moving, so you can't look back at the scene to figure out how well you noted what was there. However, you can give yourself a subjective rating about how well you were able to recall what you observed. How much detail were you able to see in the playback? Then, notice how well you are doing each time you do this. Generally, you will find you feel increasingly comfortable about doing this and recall more as you get used to the technique.

I am an Audio Recorder

In this technique, you imagine that you are a tape recorder or a cassette recorder and try to encode and recall in as much detail as you can. It's a technique that works well when you are mainly listening to something rather than viewing it, such as when you are listening to a radio talk show, lecture, or phone conversation.

In this case, imagine that you have turned yourself on as the recorder and are recording whatever you are listening to. If there is a visual image, such as a professor giving a class or speaker doing a presentation, only look at that if it enhances the audio recording you are making of what the person is saying. For example, there may be gestures and facial expressions that relate to the message. But your focus should be on the audio message.

Keep the recording going for as long as you can pay careful attention. If you find your attention wandering, put the recorder on pause; rest your mind for 5 to 10 minutes; then resume listening carefully. When you feel you have recorded enough— or feel you can't concentrate well anymore—stop the process.

Again, you can't test yourself precisely, since you are listening to words that are continually changing; there is no way to actually capture those words. But as with the video camera technique, you can give yourself a subjective rating—in this case, rate how well you were able to recall what you heard. Ask yourself, "How much detail was I able to recall the playback?"

Again, notice how you are doing each time you do this. Generally, you will feel increasingly comfortable doing this and you will recall more—and recall it more accurately, too.

Charting Your Progress

Practice working with these different techniques and see which ones work best for you. Initially, remind yourself to start the recorder going—either by consciously reminding yourself or by using the trigger that we mentioned at the beginning of the chapter. In time, you will find the reaction becomes automatic. Whenever you see or hear something that you want to pay closer attention to, the camera or recorder in your mind will immediately kick in and start recording.

A good way to chart your progress is to notice how much more you are able to remember about something you have observed or heard when you have the recorder on versus when it is off. In addition, notice how much more you are able to record as you continue to use this technique. To chart the difference, rate your experience of your ability to remember from 1 (not so good) to 5 (doing great).

24

Record and Replay

Have you ever had the experience of trying to remember where you placed your keys, where you left your car, or where you left that all-important briefcase or document? Have you ever tried to remember who you spoke to about what, where?

Such experiences are quite common. They happen to everyone, and they don't usually portend the onset of a serious memory disorder like Alzheimer's. But with these memory techniques, you will experience fewer of these lapses or will be able to more quickly recall where you left something or what happened where.

Record It Well

The first step to remembering past events is to be more attentive and in the present when these events occur, as discussed in Chapter 5 on paying attention. You have to be more mindful, and a good way to do this is to remind yourself, such as through self-talk, that you now have to be on high alert and pay attention. Stop for a moment to more fully scan and take in where you are and what you are experiencing. Then, as discussed in other chapters, use various techniques to make a good recording, such as:

- Imagine yourself a still or video camera to vividly record a series of shots of what you are seeing (Chapter 23).

- Repeat and rehearse any names, from people to street signs to your floor and row number in a parking lot (Chapter 14).

- Think about how what you are observing or who you are talking to can be of benefit to you, using the self-referent technique (Chapter 9).

The advantage of using these initial steps is that you create a stronger memory trace when you record this information. Then you are better able to access that memory later.

Play It Again, Sam!

But what if you can't immediately retrieve a memory of an event or experience after the fact? A good way to retrieve it is by putting yourself back mentally—or even physically—in the place where the event or experience occurred. Then, in your mind's eye, see yourself re-experiencing what happened. As best you can, put yourself back in time and *experience* yourself there

While this replay technique works well when you are physically in the spot where the event occurred—such as when you are in the parking lot trying to figure out where you parked your car or you are in the house where you left your keys—this technique can also make for a very strong experience if you can find a quiet place to meditate on whatever happened. Once you are there, using relaxation techniques like those described in Chapter 7, get very, very relaxed with your eyes closed, so you are totally in the moment. Let the experience come back to you and move through it again, like it is happening NOW!

This is a technique I've used from time to time to find my car or my keys. Typically this has happened when I have been distracted by thinking about something else, so I haven't properly recorded the event in the first place. Has that ever happened to you? Then, when I have returned, I suddenly see the vast parking lot stretching out ahead of me without a clue as to where my car is. Or I walk to the bowl in the hall where I typically leave my keys, find that they are not there, and have no idea where to go next. Do you know the feeling?

However, I have found that imagining myself back in time—to when I first arrived at the parking lot or first came into the house—and letting my intuitive or unconscious mind take over has retrieved the memory. I have literally seen myself driving the car into the parking lot, driving down some rows, and parking. I have seen myself walking into my house while holding my keys and walking through some rooms until I have put them down. Then, back in the present, I know where to go to find the car or keys.

In some cases, when you start this technique, you may not even see yourself retracing your steps from the past. Instead, your intuition will kick in, and suddenly you may feel drawn to the place where you left whatever you are looking for.

It helps if you can be physically in the place where the event occurred when you try to play it backwards to remember what happened. In fact, this is a technique that the police use when they are trying to get a witness to remember what happened and they physically escort the witness to that place. Once the witness is positioned where he or she originally witnessed the event—or as close to that site as possible—the cops ask questions about what the witness saw, heard, or experienced. Being back in the setting triggers cues for the witness that aid in memory recall.

The reason being back in the place where the memory was created helps is because of the power of context in remembering. This is what cognitive psychologists call the "encoding specificity principle," which states: "recall is better if the retrieval context is similar to the encoding context."[1] Another term psychologists use for this phenomenon is "context-dependent memory." In other words, if you first learn or experience something somewhere, you will better remember if you are back in the same place. Then, once you are there, imagine you are back when the event or experience occurred, and let your intuition or unconscious guide you by bringing back the memories triggered by the setting—or by guiding you to where you want to be.

Using the Replay Two-Step

You might try this replay technique using a two-step process. First, try just visualizing what happened in your mind, going through the route you took or the chronology of events you did to evoke that memory. Sometimes that may be all you need to recall what you want.

Sometimes, however, visualizing is not enough. The second step, then, is to go back to the site where the route or sequence of events started. Often, going back to that place will trigger your memories. Sometimes being there will put you back in that frame of mind, or you may see other things on the site that will trigger your recall, too.

For example, when you first confront a vast parking lot and don't recall where you parked your car, one approach is to visualize yourself driving in and through the lot. Or go to the lot and stand at the entrance. Then, as best you can, retrace your original route. As you do, let your unconscious guide you. You may not have been aware consciously as you were driving because you were driving on automatic, but your unconscious may have been taking in information about where you were. So consciously, you may not know, but your unconscious knows.

I've had this experience myself many times. For example, a number of times I've gone to an event in an area where I have been before, and thinking about getting to the event, I've parked the car without mindfully noting where I am. Then, when I leave the event, I suddenly wonder: "Where is the car?" I might not easily be able to recall where it is if I try to think about the location consciously, because I have parked in the area on different streets many times before. But when I relax and experience myself driving earlier that night, suddenly the realization of where the car is comes back. Obviously, it's best to remind yourself when arriving to pay attention and note such things as the cross-streets where you have parked. But if you don't, let your unconscious do the walking—either in your mind or let it guide you as you physically walk to where your unconscious is leading. I've used both steps of this process—individually or in sequence—to locate keys, papers, and other objects in the house when I have put them down somewhere without thinking about what I was doing. Generally it is best to have a specific location where you keep important things you use, such as keys. But even when you do, sometimes you might get distracted—say the phone rings as you are coming in the garage door with some packages and you drop the keys on a kitchen counter or by the phone. Turning the search over to your unconscious can help you make a beeline to wherever you have put something down, as I have found again and again.

What Do You Want to Recall?

Besides locating misplaced or lost objects or recalling crime events, this replay technique works well for many other situations when you want to retrieve a memory from your past experience, such as recalling:

- A conversation you had with someone, so you recall not only who it was with, but what was said
- An interview with a person for a report or article
- What happened at a meeting or water cooler conversation
- A route to a place you have been before
- A conflict or argument you had with someone
- A great party you attended
- A moment in the past you want to re-experience, such as catching that big fish and winning first prize for it
- The procedure you followed to learn a skill or perform some activity
- What happened to you as a child or teenager in your long-ago past
- A scene from a movie that moved you
- How a speaker or teacher demonstrated some subject or idea

This technique works best when it is anchored to some experiences or events that you can see or imagine vividly in your mind's eye. It doesn't work well if you are trying to recall a lot of theoretical, abstract, or factual information, where techniques like the Loci or

Roman Room methods or self-referential techniques are more appropriate. The reason it works best with concrete images or experiences is that you are essentially creating photos or movies in your mind that you play back to retrieve.

Keeping It Light

The purpose of the replay technique is to bring back a past experience to get information you need now. However, at times, you may find you are recalling strong emotional feelings about something. If you find that you are suddenly dredging up emotionally charged memories, such as in trying to replay incidents from your childhood or a messy conflict with a former friend or lover, stop the process by opening your eyes or turning your attention to something else. You don't want to delve into something heavy right now. Push such feelings away or turn away from them now.

But it may be a good idea to recognize and deal with such feelings at a later time when you can deal with them appropriately. For example, if you find that you are tapping into heavy emotions, this might be something to go over and work on with a counselor, therapist, or supportive friend or family member. This way you don't try to suppress anything that could be important to you, but you deal with it at another time in a more appropriate way, and do so in a supportive environment that can help you deal with it.

Going Even Deeper

While using your imagination generally works for everyday situations, like finding lost objects, recalling what happened at a meeting, and remembering what happened at that party last night, it is possible to go deeper and bring up less-accessed or long-buried memories. This can be useful for such things as recalling what you liked to do in high school or college, deciding on a career change, or remembering details of an incident for a court case. But to deal with serious personal issues that are emotionally charged, don't use this technique on your own. Instead do this in a controlled, supportive setting, such as with a trained hypnotist or counselor.

The basic approach for going deeper is to get in a relaxed, meditative state in a quiet place, where you can tap into your inner self, unconscious, or intuition. Start by using a relaxation technique to get very, very relaxed, though your mind remains alert. Then, ask yourself a series of questions about what you want to remember; and after that let your inner self take over to guide the process. Think of this process as taking a journey back into your past, where you will experience being there, so you will recall what you observed, heard, taste, smelled, and felt at the time.

Following is an example of a guided journey you might use. Plug in your own questions. You can tape this and play it back while you listen and take the trip back into your memory. Or read this to give you a general guide; then give yourself the instructions mentally, before turning it over to your inner consciousness. Reflect on your experience immediately after you return to normal consciousness. To further aid your recall, write down what you experienced, so you can review it for further insights later.

> *Start by getting very relaxed. Begin by paying attention to your breathing. Notice your breath going in and out, in and out. You are feeling more and more relaxed; more and more relaxed.*
>
> *Now imagine that you are going back in time to when you were a certain age or when this incident happened. Just experience yourself going back in time, going back, going back, to whenever and wherever you want to be.*
>
> *Now you are there. Look around and notice what's there. Notice the environment around you. Are you in the country, in the city, in a building? Wherever you are, take some time to just experience being there.*
>
> *Now ask yourself questions that you would like to answer from this trip back in time. You can see these questions appear on a screen in front of you or just hear them in your mind. Just ask the first question, and then listen and observe. What do you see? Hear? Take a minute or two to do this.*
>
> *Now ask your next question. Again, just listen and observe. Notice what you see. Pay attention to what you hear. Again, take a minute or two to do this.*

Now ask any additional questions. Go through the same process of listening and observing.

Finally, when you are finished asking your questions, return to the room and your normal consciousness. Count backwards from five to one; five, four. Getting more and more alert. Three, two. More and more alert and awake. One, you are back in the room.

Once you are back, reflect on what you experienced and learned. Write it down to help solidify what you discovered on your journey into your memory.

Practice the Technique

Take some time now to practice with these techniques. Even if there's nothing you are trying to remember right now, try out each of these techniques as follows:

1. Pick out something that has happened recently that you haven't thought about for awhile—such as a meeting at work, a conversation with a friend. Then, focus your attention on that event and visualize it in your mind. Don't pay attention to any outside distractions; consider using earplugs if you are doing this in an area that's noisy, such as a busy office with keyboards clicking and phones ringing. You might think of yourself like a film director on a set watching a movie unfold in front of you. Start at the beginning of the event or incident and watch it unfold in front of you. Make your visualization of this event as vivid as possible. Notice the environment around you, the sounds you hear, and observe what happens. Listen to what is being said in a conversation or meeting. Be as complete as possible.

Then, write down the highlights of what you remember. Pay attention to your experience of remembering, too, and later, when you do this exercise again, compare it to your previous experience with this technique. You will generally find that your ability to do this and remember will improve.

2. Now using the same event or another event, go to the actual location where it occurred. Pick an event that occurred in a con-

tained and easily accessible location, such as a room in your home or building in your community, so you can walk through this location. Of course, you can use this technique with distant or multiple locations, too (as sometimes occurs in a court case when witnesses are taken to different locations). Start from where the event occurred, and if the incident involved moving from one place to another (such as driving your car into town or walking from room to room), do that, too. As you stand or sit at the beginning of this event, look around you first and then go through the same visualization process as above. Observe and experience whatever is around you with great concentration and make your visualization of this event as vivid as possible. Both in reality and in your mind's eye, notice the environment around you, the sounds you hear, and observe what happens. Then, if you moved through this location during the event, walk through the same route, being attentive to any triggering cues in your environment, as well as calling up what happened in that location in the past. Be as complete as possible.

Then, write down the highlights of what you remember. Pay attention to your experience of remembering, too, and compare this experience to what happened when you tried to remember using your power of visualization only. Commonly, your experience will be even more vivid when you are actually there, because of the triggering power of contextual cues.

If you chose the same event as in the previous exercise, your previous recollections of this event should help you in recalling what happened. But at the same time, you should notice even more, so if there were any gaps in your memory in the first go-around, you will likely be able to fill them in.

Later, when you do this real-world replay process again, compare it to your previous real-world replay experience. You will generally find that your ability to do this and remember will improve.

3. Finally, try the deeper recall process. Pick some past event you would like to remember. Keep it to a business or leisure time event, so you can experience it very vividly, but without a lot of emotional content. For example, this is not the time to go back over a messy divorce, an ugly battle with a significant other, or other experience

with negative baggage. You want something that will be light and fun to remember.

Then, find a quiet, comfortable place where you can get relaxed and use the guidelines provided above to guide you into the experience. Once you are there, notice everything around you—the sights, the sounds, the smells, the tastes, and let yourself go on the journey, as you remember what it was like to be there at the time.

Experience this for about 5–15 minutes. Afterward, reflect on the experience and write down the highlights. Later, when you try this again, notice what the experience was like each time. Generally, you will find it easier and easier to go back and remember, and will remember more.

25

Body Language

You may have heard the old song about "dem bones"—the leg bone's connected to the thigh bone, the thigh bone's connected to the hip bone, the hip bone's connected to the . . . and so on, until you end up with the head bone. Well, the body system for remembering short lists is something like that. You start with your foot and go up your body until you come to the hair on your head (or your bald pate if you don't have any hair). Or you could go in the opposite direction, starting with your head. It's essentially a number system, except you use your body—preferably for up to 10 items, though you could add more to your list by adding more body parts.

As in other association systems, you simply associate strong visual images for what you want to remember with that body part.

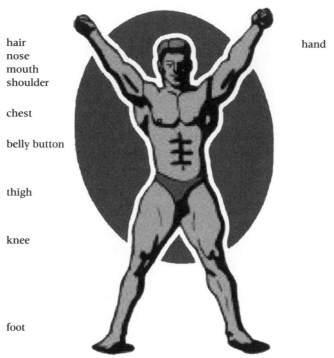

hair
nose
mouth
shoulder

chest

belly button

thigh

knee

foot

hand

Using Your Body to Learn Short Lists

You can pick any body parts you prefer, but here's how it would work if you have a shopping list with these items: glue, cat food, broccoli, chicken, grapes, sour cream, toothpaste, vitamins, orange juice, and CD disks. Starting at your foot, you might create the following image associations:

- Your **foot** is stuck in a pot of **glue.**
- A hungry cat is jumping on your **knee** looking for **cat food**.
- A stalk of **broccoli** is sticking out of your pants pocket on your **thigh.**
- A **chicken** is pecking at your **belly button.**
- A bunch of **grapes** are hanging from your **chest.**
- Your sore **shoulders** are being rubbed by **sour cream.**
- You have a toothbrush with **toothpaste** on it sticking out of your **mouth.**

- You have **vitamin pills** pasted onto your **nose.**
- Your **hair** is covered with shiny **orange juice.**
- You are holding several **CD disks** in your **hand.**

That's how it works. Now here's a list of items for you to try associating with different parts of your body. After you come up with a series of images, go over them in your mind. Then, close the book, and see how many you can remember on your own body. Afterwards, try creating your own shopping lists. Or play the Body Parts Game with some friends and have fun sharpening your memory—you could even call it an out-of-body experience!

Here's your list to remember. You can connect the items with any body part.

BODY PARTS AND LIST TO REMEMBER	
Camera	
Milk	
Eggs	
Shampoo	
Candy	
Lettuce	
Tomatoes	
Coffee	
Honey	
Soap	

Now create your own list here:

BODY PARTS AND LIST TO REMEMBER	

Playing the Body Parts Game

Play with at least three people. In turn, each person creates a list of any type—from a shopping list to objects in the office—and describes his or her body associations with those items. Then, the other players try to list as many of the items in that list as possible and announce when their list is completed by calling out, "Got it." The person with the longest list wins—or if there is a tie, the first person to call "Got it" wins.

As you play this game, your ability to imagine connections and remember lists should improve, too.

26

Let Your Intuition Do the Walking

Memory systems can be great, but sometimes turning recall over to your intuition is what you need to recapture a memory for something that happened in the immediate past or long ago. Using your intuition can even help you recapture a dream or remember what you said in a conversation with someone.

I had several such experiences myself while writing this book.

In one case, I had been using some files for my August bills and income receipts, and afterwards I sent out some letters using preprinted return addresses, which I kept in several other files on my desk. A few days later, I went to the file cabinet where I keep my bills and receipts, but the August files weren't there—and when I looked in all the logical places in the room and several other rooms, they weren't there either. So I tried to reconstruct everything I did or might have done using those files, from making phone calls to paying bills, but nothing seemed to work. I even looked several times through the file cabinet where the files should have been, thinking maybe I might have misplaced them in the wrong order. But that didn't work either. They were simply gone.

Feeling very frustrated, I let go of my thinking mind, asked the question to myself, "Where did I go?" as if I were that file, and walked through my house, giving myself over to my experience in each room. Suddenly, as I came to the file cabinet, I felt drawn to a small rack of shelves beside the file cabinet, where I had put the file for preprinted return addresses, and picked it up. And there at the bottom of the stack were my two file folders of August bills and income received. Memory accomplished. I hadn't used conscious thinking or any particular image system. I just gave the task over to my unconscious, which drew on its own traces of memory, which were out of my awareness, to lead me to pick up the files in the rack of shelves, where I had inadvertently put the August files.

Another time, I had left my car in a large parking garage with several levels. I was in a rush to get some books and papers onto a wheeled cart so I could get to a meeting. As a result, I forgot to do the usual techniques to imprint where I was parked in my memory, including looking at the sign with the letter and number of my section of the lot. So when I came back and saw a sea of cars, the task of finding my car seemed daunting. But then, intuition came once again to the rescue. I stopped thinking consciously about where I had parked the car; I stopped trying to create mental maps and reconstruct where I had gone as I drove into the parking lot. Instead, I let my intuition take over. Without thinking about where I was going, I walked back to the car, letting my mind unconsciously backtrack how I had walked out of the parking garage to my meeting.

I also used this approach to think about some of my earliest memories by projecting myself back into my childhood when I was about four or five. It was like I was right there again, recalling one of my very first memories of being at a large train station, crossing the tracks, and feeling awed by the vastness of it all, as I walked quickly to keep up with my mother who had taken me on a trip to Florida by train to see my grandmother. (Those were the days before people normally went to airports to take planes.)

Finally, I used this intuitive approach to recapture a dream, where I had only the sense that I had been dreaming and a fleeting image of what had been the end of the dream, before it slipped away, like a stealthy jaguar, going back to hiding in the jungle. Consciously, I couldn't seem to pull the dream out by that last image; I couldn't pull on the tail of the jaguar to tease it out. Instead, I relaxed with that last possible image in mind, projecting myself back into that dream state I had been in. Suddenly, I was there, re-experiencing the dream again, and a few minutes later, when I opened my eyes, the dream was in my mind, letting me record it before it flitted away again out of my working memory, unlikely to be recalled again. Dreams often do not go into long-term memory once they are gone; unless you do something to preserve those images, they normally slip away for good.

How and Why the Intuitive Process Works

Certainly, any kind of memory process will work better, including tapping into your unconscious, when you have made a clear impression of something. That's because the memory trace is brighter, louder, or otherwise more intense, so you can see, hear, or experience it better. But even if you have only imprinted something slightly or the trace has faded, these intuitive techniques can help you dig back into the more flimsy impressions in your unconscious to retrieve information.

A good way to think of this process is to recognize that every impression, every sensation, no matter how minor, makes some kind of imprint on the neurons in your brain. Researchers have found that this is the case by tapping certain parts of the brain, using special probes to trigger certain memories. Also, they use the PET (positron emission tomography) scan technique to show which areas of the brain are activated when you perform different memory tasks.

As a result, researchers believe that all impressions that create memories can be found somewhere within the brain. In other words, every image we see, every sound or conversation we hear, every experience we have that gets transferred into our long-term memory from our working memory gets registered someplace in the brain. Although many of these memories fade from consciousness and many are just lightly recorded, they are there, somewhere, though other experiences that leave little impression may not get transferred. That's why certain processes, like hypnosis and deep concentration, as well as certain physical stimuli, can pull the memories that do get transferred back. The less clear, more faded impressions will be harder to tap, since they are so much fainter. But they are still there. While some researchers may claim that all experiences are registered, others suggest it is just the experiences that become part of the working memory. Perhaps consider the process like traveling on a bus. Some memories will go to the end of the line—into the working memory—where they get recorded and the record is there to be retrieved later, but others get off early on—like everyday working memories, and after they slip off, they are gone forever.

In turn, a good way to trigger the recall of a memory is to try to go back to or recreate the time when you first created that impression in your brain cells. This return—along with your intense focus—helps to evoke the event or setting that will remind you of the memory and pull it into the present. This approach works because it's like making the memory live again; it's like finding a book you really find involving. You open up the book and as you read it, you project yourself back into the pages, so you actually experience what's on that page. Instead of just an abstract, detached perception of what is there, you are reliving the experience; you are making that page, which is like your memory, come alive; you are making it more intensely, vividly real.

For example, to recall a name, imagine the person before you, perhaps at your first meeting. To recall a phone number, visualize a time when you looked up the number in a book, wrote it down on a piece of paper, or dialed it. To recall where you put some object, imagine yourself in the situation where you last had that object and notice what you did with it when you put it down. To recall a route, imagine yourself in the car or on foot traveling along it from where you started. To recall some information from a book or movie, visualize yourself reading the book or watching the film. To recall what happened at an event or in a particular situation, imagine yourself there as vividly as possible and play out the scene in your mind.

Don't try to think about what you are experiencing; just be in a very receptive state where you experience and feel and let your unconscious bring the memory back to you. It's as if you are letting your unconscious talk to you, paint a picture, or write a script for you in your mind's eye, while you just watch, listen, and experience what is happening, like a spectator in an audience.

In short, the key to recalling things when you have trouble doing so is to trigger your unconscious to bring the memory to you. You start the process by getting into a very relaxed, meditative state, in which you see the scene by drawing on as many of your senses as possible, so you recreate the original experience to feel yourself actually there. Then, it's not like you are trying to remember something that once happened. Rather, with the help of your unconscious or intuition, you are seeing and experiencing that incident now, so you can recall through re-creation and re-experiencing it, much more than you otherwise could.

Tapping into Your Unconscious Powers

There are varying ways to tap into your intuition. These techniques help you release your unconscious processes, so you can dig back into the inner storage area in your unconscious to retrieve it.

Whether you want to recover a name, a telephone number, the location of an object, a route you traveled, or whatever, to recall it you must recreate the original experience in your mind as realistically and dramatically as possible. If you're in a setting where you can replay the experience in reality, do it. That will help you recapture the memory.

When you first try doing this technique, you might do some preparation to get you in an alternative dreamy or meditative state of mind. Use a relaxation technique, such as described in Chapter 7, to get in this altered state, but not so relaxed that you fall asleep. The hynogogic and hypnopompic states, when you are drifting off to sleep or first wake up and are only partially conscious but not asleep, are other examples of the kind of state to be in to release your unconscious. Thus, if you don't fully rouse yourself in the morning when you first wake up, you may be able to recapture that dream.

When you get accustomed to using this technique, you can do it anywhere. You don't even need to close your eyes. You can simply focus on releasing your conscious mind; then focus on your inner mental screen and see the image there before you or listen to your internal tape or CD player. Just be receptive and let the image or sounds flow into your mind.

While you can will yourself to go back in time to re-experience a particular event, whether in recent times or in your long-ago past, it helps if you can put yourself in the actual setting—as I did when I was by the file cabinet, and I suddenly felt drawn to pick up some files. Similarly, being in the parking lot at the spot where I had originally left my car to go to the meeting helped to pull me back, so I was able to unconsciously retrace my steps.

When you first start using this method, don't expect to have instant recall right away. Take a few minutes to settle down and visualize yourself in the setting. After a while, with practice, the process becomes much faster, so you will soon be able to retrieve a memory within moments.

The following recall techniques will help you remember names, phone numbers, where you put an object, a route you traveled, or something you read or saw in a movie. Also, these techniques will help you recall situations and events. Plan to practice each one for a few days. Then, after you feel comfortable with the technique, you can use it as needed. Begin practicing each technique by getting relaxed and closing your eyes. Later, you'll find you can do it without closing your eyes.

Consider these techniques supplements to anything else you might do to remember, such as rehearsal and chunking. Basically, they all work by helping you return to the situation where you first engaged in a particular activity, whether or not you consciously did anything to encode the experience in memory at that time. Then, once you return to the original scene in your mind or by physically going there, you let go of your conscious mind and let your unconscious pull out whatever you have unconsciously recorded in your unconscious mind.

Recalling a Name

This technique will help you recall the name you are trying to remember.

> *Visualize the person before you. Imagine that you are meeting for the first time, and review this first meeting very closely. Be aware of who else is there, the setting, and so on. Make your picture as complete as possible.*

Then, greet this person as you did when you first met, and listen carefully as he or she tells you his or her name.

Recalling a Phone Number

This technique, similar to the one above, should help you retrieve the phone number you need.

Visualize a telephone before you and see the person you are going to call near a phone, awaiting your call.

Now imagine you are opening your telephone book or computer calendar to the name of this person. The number will often appear, but if it seems hazy, begin dialing the number, and as you dial, the number will become clear.

Alternatively, if you have recently written down the person's number, visualize yourself in that situation. The person is telling you his or her number and you are writing it down. Notice the setting where you are. Be aware of the type of paper you are using to write your note. Then, see yourself writing the number and repeat it to yourself as you write it. The number will appear clearly before you and you will remember it.

Recalling Where You Put an Object

This will help you find the item you are looking for.

Think back to the last time you had that object. Where were you? What were you doing with it? Visualize yourself using that object. Then, when you are finished with it, observe what you do with it when you put it away.

Recalling a Route

And they say you can't go home again!

Visualize yourself in a car or on foot, as in your original experience. Don't try to retrace your steps backwards, but begin where you started. Now see yourself leaving from this starting point. Be aware of the surroundings you pass. Notice how far you go and look for significant route markers or landmarks. Speed up on straightaways, and pay careful attention to what is around you when you make a turn. Keep going until you get to your destination.

Recalling Information from a Book

This is not a technique for studying and is certainly not meant to replace your regular study routines (chunk, categorize, rehearse, review, and repeat). However, it can help you retrieve information from a book or article that you were casually reading.

Visualize yourself reading the book. Hold it in your hands and feel it there—be aware of its size, shape, and texture. If it was an article in a magazine, remember what was on the cover, feel the glossy pages, smell that special magazine-y smell.

Begin turning pages, until you get to the page you want. Then, look down the page to the appropriate paragraph or line and read.

Recalling a Scene from a Movie

This will help you recall a scene you saw in a movie.

Experience being at the movie as intensely as possible. Sense the darkness around you; sink down in your seat; smell and taste the popcorn.

When the movie comes on the screen, see the title vividly, and fast-forward the film to what you want to recall.

Then, slow the projector to normal speed again and watch the scene unfold that you want to see. Watch the characters act and converse just as you did at the movie itself, and you'll see the movie again vividly in your mind.

Recalling a Situation or Event

Aren't you lucky! A movie was made of that very situation—and you were the director. Watch the daily rushes.

Imagine yourself in the situation as vividly as possible. Notice the setting, the buildings, the people around you. Imagine you are a movie director and this is a scene that is about to unfold before you. You hold the script in your hands, and at your cue, the actors in the situation begin to play out the scene. You are able to notice everything, hear everything they say.

If you want to move ahead faster in the scene, simply turn a page of your script, say "cut," and direct the actors to start again in a later scene.

Once you have gained practice in recalling the memories you want with these techniques, feel free to develop your own imagery to help you recall any situation or event. For example, you may see yourself as an investigative reporter covering a story rather than a movie director filming a script.

The key to recall is to imagine yourself as vividly as possible in the situation you want to remember. Then, you use your mental picture or recording of that situation to stimulate your unconscious memory of the original event.

27

Remembering Names and Faces

One of the biggest reasons for wanting to improve your memory is to better remember names and faces. It's something that people who deal with the public—such as salespeople and politicians—are particularly concerned about, and it often can make the difference between getting the sale or the vote . . . or not. After all, when you remember someone's name—and can further personalize that by what you remember about that person—he or she is flattered; people feel appreciative that you remembered them. And that can translate into votes, sales, gaining customers, getting referrals, and more.

So let's start with remembering names; then faces; and finally making further associations with facts about the person.

Remembering Names

Here are specific ways to apply the techniques you have already learned earlier to remember names.

Pay Attention

A first step is to pay attention when you meet someone, so you listen to the name and observe the person's face. In fact, one of the main reasons for forgetting a name is that you haven't paid attention to learning it in the first place. You know the common experience. You are distracted during introductions, are thinking about making a good impression, or are looking around the room for someone you are supposed to meet with, or something else. You have already met a dozen people and your mind glazes over as you meet someone new.

It doesn't matter how many others you have already met—you must remind yourself to be alert and focus on the person you are meeting. Use a mental trigger word or a physical trigger to give yourself a mental tug to be present in the room. And if you don't catch the person's name the first time, don't feel embarrassed about asking the person to repeat it. Generally, people will be flattered by your show of interest in asking them to repeat their name so you get it right.

Repeat and Rehearse

Beyond just hearing the name, repeat it to yourself mentally and try to repeat it in conversation. That way you will transfer the name from your working to your long-term memory. Additionally, if you say the name aloud in conversation, that will assure you that you heard the name correctly—and if not, the person will likely correct you. But in saying the name aloud, don't overdo it; you don't want to sound like a broken record. Two or three times is fine, and if you are saying good-night or good-bye, use the name as you leave, too.

Mention Anything Special about the Name

If you notice anything unusual or outstanding about the name, or if it reminds you of someone or something you know, mention it. If it's appropriate, say your observation about the name aloud, such as saying something like: "Oh, a Coddington was a member of our City Council." Or if you are unable to mention something special—such as when you only briefly meet a number of people—just repeat that odd fact mentally to yourself.

Create a Visual or Mental Association with the Name

Creating a visual or mental association, just like in remembering any list of items, will make the name come alive. There are three ways to create this visual or mental association with different types of names.

- If the name already has a meaning, such as Fox, Baker, Carpenter, or Brown, use that, such as seeing Jim Fox as a sly fox working out on equipment in a gym, or seeing Carol Baker as a woman who is singing Christmas carols while she bakes.

- If the name doesn't immediately have a meaning, as is true of most names, see if you can come up with other meaningful associations. For example, if the person's name is Washington, you might think of President George Washington; if the person's name is Jordan, you might think of the basketball player Michael Jordan or the river Jordan.

- If the name has no meaning, you can use the substitute words technique, described in Chapter 21, to break down the word into a substitute word or idea. For example, if you meet a Mr. Wallace, you might think of a "wall" and the "ace" in a card deck; if you meet Joyce Granger, you might think of a woman jumping with "joy" on a boat at "sea," and then think of a park "ranger" with a large "G" on his jacket. Just think of whatever first comes to mind. As memory expert Harry Lorayne points out in *How to Develop a Super Power Memory*,[1] you don't have to use a substitute that sounds exactly like the name or use words for every part of the name. That's because "if you remember the main (idea), the incidentals will fall into place by true memory."

To remember titles, such as Dr. or Ph.D., use an additional mental image, such as seeing the person holding a stethoscope for a doctor, or seeing a small crawling bug (an a**Phid)** for the Ph.D.

Clarify How the Person Wants to Be Called

If appropriate, you can ask what the person prefers being called, such as when a person with a longer name like "William" or "Gwendolyn" might prefer to be called Bill or Gwen. This question might be particularly appropriate if you are being introduced to the person by someone else and start talking. In many cases, people will use both names interchangeably, but prefer the shorter version in an informal situation, like a party or social networking event. In some cases, if this is an unfamiliar or unusual name, you might ask how the person spells the name, too.

Make the Name Meaningful to You

Remember the self-referent effect described in Chapter 9? Well, that approach can work in remembering names, particularly as you learn more about the person. One strategy is to think about other people you know well who have the same name. Another is to think about how knowing the person will be important to you—for example, is the person a likely customer or client for certain products or services, is there some activity you would like to do with the person, do you know someone in common? The link to you will help the person's name stand out in your mind.

Get a Business Card

You can always use a memory aid to help you, too, particularly if you are getting a lot of names at the same time, such as at a networking event or trade show. There may not be time to encode everyone's name in your memory with creative associations and meaningful connections to yourself. Or you may not be able to repeat a person's name in a few seconds of conversation. In that case, simply get a card. To distinguish the reason for contacting this person later from all the other cards you have collected, write a brief note on the front or back of the card about what to do (such as: "call about getting flowers"). Then, file the cards you have collected, by event, and review your cards shortly afterwards, so you can repeat the name to yourself as well as remember why you took that person's card and what to do.

Reflect and Review

When you leave the place or event where you have met a person, reflect back and try to recall the names of all the people you have met. Say their names aloud. Write down their names on a list as soon as you get a chance. And as you recall their names, think about what they looked like. You might even talk about the people you met with other people.

Use the 4-Point SALT Method

Finally, you might use the 4-Point SALT method suggested by memory expert Douglas J. Herrmann[2]:

1. **Say** the name out loud.
2. **Ask** the person a question using his or her name.
3. **(At) Least** once, use the name in conversation.
4. **Terminate** the conversation by using the name again.

Remembering Faces

Remembering the name won't do you much good if you attach it to the wrong face. Here are specific ways and techniques to remember faces.

Notice Distinctive Features

Just as you need to pay attention to a person's name, you should focus on the person's face, too. Be sure to look directly at the person, and as you are being introduced, make eye contact. As you look at the person's face, carefully notice any distinctive features. To help you notice them, ask yourself questions such as: "Does he have a large or small nose?" "Are her ears large or is she wearing earrings?" "What color are his eyes?" "What is the shape of her chin?" You might even imagine yourself a police artist trying to come up with a sketch of a criminal and asking the victim to describe the suspect's distinctive traits. Or imagine what you would do if you were a cartoonist making a caricature of the person. What parts of the person's face might you exaggerate so they stand out even more? Some features that might stand out could be:

- Big or small eyes
- Thick or thin lips, wide or small mouth
- High or low forehead, smooth or creased forehead
- Long or short nose, thick or broad nose, wide or narrow nostrils
- Large or small ears, ears that stick out
- Dimples or freckles, clefts
- Warts or beauty marks, wrinkles and lines
- Large, jutting, or receding chin
- Type of hairline and hairstyle, beard or mustache
- Type of smile
- Earrings

In short, just about anything might be an outstanding or distinctive feature.

However, be careful about features that might come and go, like beards, mustaches, eyeglasses, and hairstyles. While they might be distinctive now, when you meet the person another time he or she might still not have this feature, so while you might use this as a feature that stands out now, don't make it a defining characteristic.

Notice Personal Qualities

Once you notice a distinctive quality, try to assign some characteristic to help it further stand out. For instance, besides noticing a person's blue eyes, notice how vibrant they are. If someone has a jutting chin, consider how strong that is. Also, consider how the person's face reflects what the person is like. For instance, does their face appear happy or sad? Full of energy or tired? Outgoing or shy?

Use Associations to Connect the Name and Face

Notice if anything about the person's face can be linked to their name. Here are a few examples of how this works.

- Say you meet a woman named Victoria Lyons, who has a happy face with a toothy smile. You might think of a pair of lions (Lyons) holding sexy lingerie (associated with Victoria's Secret, known for its sexy clothing designs) with their long teeth (associated with her many teeth). In short, you have created an image association that incorporates both the woman's name and her face. Then, condense that image, such as seeing a small lion perched on her head. Later, when you try to recall her name, as you think of her face, the image of the lion on her head will trigger the other associations, and voila—you will remember her name—Victoria Lyons.

- Or take this example suggested by Harry Lorayne.[3] To create an image for a Mr. Sachs who has a very high forehead, "you might see millions of sacks falling from his forehead or see his forehead as a sack instead of a forehead."
- And here's one more example from Dominic O'Brien, author of *How to Develop a Brilliant Memory Week by Week*.[4] Say you meet a man named Peter Byrd, who has a hooked nose that suggests a beak. You might associate his first name with "Pet" and his last name with "Bird," so you think of a pet bird, and to make the association even more vivid, you see the pet bird flying around in your house.

You can come up with any image you want that links the person's face and name. What's most important is that you see the image vividly in your mind's eye, so later you can call up this image to remind you of both the person's face and their name.

Find a Place for the Face

Still another face-saving—that is, remembering—technique is suggested by Dominic O'Brien, who remembers people's faces by "giving the face a place," since we tend to associate a person with a particular place.[5] It's the experience you have when you see a person whose face is familiar and the first thing you try to do is remember where you know this person from. When you think of the place, it triggers the memory of the person's name and other memories you have associated with this person. To use this technique, you associate the person with a place as soon as you meet them by imagining where you might expect to find that person.

For instance, if you meet a person who looks like a librarian, you might think of someone you know personally or otherwise (such as a politician or celebrity) with that name and imagine them working at your local library. As an example, say you meet someone named Julia; you might think of the actress Julia Roberts working at the library. Then, when you see the person's face again, it will trigger a chain of vivid associations that will pull up the name, such as in this case: face—library—Julia Roberts scene—Julia.

While this association process may seem to take a number of steps to get from the face to the name, the process happens in a quick flash, taking seconds or milliseconds. However, if the person's face has distinctive features, it may be easier to associate their name directly with their physical appearance, as in the examples above.

More Than Just a Name and Face

Remembering Information About a Person

Besides just remembering names and faces, it helps to connect additional information to that person, such as an occupation, hobbies, where the person lives, and interesting biographical tidbits. To do so, in addition to using the other techniques to remember the person's name and face, you might do any of the following:

- Repeat what the person has just told you in the conversation, such as commenting on the person's interesting occupation or hobby.

- Think about how this information relates to you and even comment on it to the person or imagine that you are saying this, such as noting that you are in a similar occupation or share the same interests.

- See a picture of the person participating in that activity, such as if Peter Byrd works at a bank, you might see him as a bird flying to work and landing behind the teller's cage—a cage for both tellers and pet birds.

Adding this information to what you remember about names and faces will help the person further come alive in your memory.

Playing the Name Game

Finally, to help you remember names, faces, and interesting information, as well as have fun doing this, you can play the Name Game
with a group of people. Here are two ways to play:

1. With a partner or in a group, cut up some pictures of unfamiliar faces from a pile of magazines or newspapers. If the pictures
don't have names, make up some first and last names. Create a set
of 7–15 pictures with names and faces, with each of you creating the
same number per set. (Start with 7; then increase the difficulty by
adding more pictures.) Swap pictures, so you each have a different
set. Now take a minute to study each of the faces before looking at
the names and concentrate on what stands out as a distinctive feature. Next, look at the names and use your imagination to create
associations. Afterwards, put the pictures aside for 10 to 15 minutes
and do something else. Then, take turns testing each other by holding up the photos and asking the other person to remember as many
names as they can for the faces in their set of photos. Score 1 point
for each correct identification, delete 1 point for each incorrect identification, and see who has the highest score.[6]

2. Collect some unfamiliar pictures of people's faces from a
magazine or newspaper and paste them on index cards or pieces of
cardboard. Make up some first and last names and put them on another set of cards. Shuffle the two sets of cards separately and turn
up a name and a face card from each of the two decks so you have
them side by side. Each person will create a series of associations for
that name and face. Then, turn that set face down.

After you go through this process 7 to 15 times (as above, start
with 7), increase the difficulty by adding one or two more sets with
additional pictures, shuffle all of the sets, and, one by one, turn up
only the face card for each set. Now it's a race to be the first person
to call out the correct name. Score 1 point for getting it correct, lose
1 point if incorrect. If the person is incorrect, keep going until someone gets it correct—or no one does. Then, go on to the next face and
name set. After you have gone through all of the sets, total the score
for each of the sets used. The player with the most points wins.

Remembering Important Numbers

If you need to remember numbers, there are a number of systems to help you do this. I don't use any of these association methods myself; I use the chunking and rehearsal methods described earlier, along with creating files for passwords and other important numbers. But numerous memory experts and authors swear by them, so I'm including the descriptions of different number systems here, along with some practice exercises. Consider these as another type of memory aid to add to your repertoire and use those that feel comfortable to you.

Turning Numbers into Sentences

This is a method where you turn each number into a word of that many letters in a sentence. As described by Dominic O'Brien in *How to Develop a Brilliant Memory Week by Week,* "each digit determines the number of letters in each word in the sequence."[1] Here's how it works. Say you want to memorize the first few places of the number pi, which is 3.1415926. You might come up with a sentence like:

HOW   I   WISH   I   COULD ENUMERATE PI EASILY
(3)   (1)   (4)   (1)   (5)   (9)   (2)   (6)

To help you connect the sentence to the number you want to remember, it's a good idea to use a sentence that relates to the number. For example, say your bank account number is 342-37842-2434; you might come up with a sentence like:

THE BANK IS THE LARGEST, GREATEST BANK IN MY CITY FOR SURE.
 (3)   (4) (2) (3)   (7)   (8)   (4) (2) (2) (4) (3)   (4)

What do you do if you have a 0? Use some punctuation symbol— like a hyphen, exclamation mark, or comma ("-" or "!" or ",")—to indicate this.

Now it's your turn. Come up with some sentences for the key numbers in your life, such as the following. Of course, if you already know the number by heart, you don't need to do this. Otherwise, write down the number and come up with a related sentence you can easily remember. If you've got a number with a lot of eights and nines in it, you may not be able to use this system. But another of the systems described here may be just the one you need.

TURNING NUMBERS INTO SENTENCES	
Number	**Sentence**
Your social security number:	
Your credit card number:	
Another credit card number:	
Your debit card number:	
Your driver's license:	
Your car's license number:	
Your bank account number:	
Your PIN card number:	
The combination for a lock or safe:	
Your e-mail password:	
Another password:	

A mortgage or loan number:	
A friend's phone number:	
Any other number:	

Keep going as long as you have numbers you want to remember. When you learn new numbers, you can add these to your memory bank for numbers too.

As long as you access these sentences fairly regularly, they will generally be easier to remember than the numbers and will remind you what the number is as soon as you say them. But just in case, for backup, you can write down the sentences, much like you might keep a list of important numbers and store it in a secure place. You want to keep this list secure, since this is an easy code to break, once someone figures out that the number of letters in each word is the key to the digits in that number.

Playing the Number Sentences Game

You can turn this process into a fun game, in which you come up with a list of random numbers. Then, players race to come up with a grammatically correct sentence the fastest.

Start with a smaller number of digits to start—say, or six or seven digits in a sequence. Then, expand the number of digits to 8, 9, 10, and finally up to 16 digits (the number of digits in a credit card).

To generate numbers, players can take turns writing a series of random numbers on a card, then turn up one of the cards. Or create a small deck of numbers, shuffle the deck, and lay out the desired number of cards in a sequence.

Once the card is turned up or all the numbers are out, the race is on. Be the first to come up with a correct sentence; stop play by calling out "Got it!" or ring a bell. Then if you are correct, score 1 point; or lose 1 point for an incorrect sentence. The next person to claim a sentence scores in the same way. The winner is the player with the most points after a series of rounds of play—or the first to score a certain number of points, such as 5 points for four players.

Use a smaller total for more players, a larger total for two or three players.

Using the Number Shapes System

Another way of remembering numbers is the "number shapes" system. This is considered a type of "peg" memory system. The way a peg system works is that you have a list of memory key images that don't change, which you use to link and associate anything you want to remember. As memory book author Tony Buzan describes it,[2] you might think of a peg system as a wardrobe with a certain number of hangers where you hang your clothes. While the clothes you hang on these hangers can change, the hangers themselves stay the same. In the number shapes system, you use numbers and shapes to represent the hangers, and you hang what you want to remember, like clothes in your wardrobe, on the hangers.

It's a fairly simple system, since you only use the numbers from 0–9 and you associate an image with each of the numbers. What makes the association easier is that the image associated with each number has the same approximate shape. You can use any of the commonly used images for a particular number, such as the "swan" for number 2, since that number is shaped like a swan. Or when you think of the number 8, a common image association is a snowman or hourglass.[3]

You can also come up with your own image. Whatever you use has to be a strong visual image that will stick in your memory. You then combine the images together for different numbers to create a strong association. The combined imagery can be as wild and crazy as you want; the idea is to have a memorable association.

For instance, to use an example from Dominic O'Brien in *How to Develop a Perfect Memory: Week by Week,* suppose you associate an elephant's trunk with the number 6 and a boomerang with the number 7. If you have a 67 bus to catch, you might imagine that the elephant is standing by the bus holding a boomerang in its trunk. Though it may be an unusual and bizarre image, it is very memorable. As O'Brien notes: "Now, suddenly, numbers come to life. They become animated, take on a unique significance and are instantly more memorable."[4]

Or say your association with number 6 is a pipe and with 7 is a fishing line. You might imagine a fisherman who is fishing and he pulls up a pipe on his fishing line. Or he is using a pipe as a fishing pole with his fishing line attached.

In the case of a bigger number, you create a longer chain of associations with the images linked to each number. Say you are trying to remember your bank PIN number, which is 4298—and your associations for each of these numbers, respectively, is a sailboat (4), a swan (2), a tennis racket (9), and a snowman (8). You might imagine that you are out sailing when you see a swan in the water, which suddenly tries to attack you, so you swat it with a tennis racquet and it turns into a snowman. A strange image, but certainly memorable!

Just use your imagination to create the associations, starting with the images you choose to represent each number. This system works because it's easier to remember the associated imagery than the number. Just be sure that you know what associations go with what number, perhaps by adding some connection to the story. For instance, in the sailboat story above, you might see yourself going to your sailboat upon leaving the bank, which reminds you that this association is for your bank PIN number. Likewise, if you create a sequence of images for your bank account number, you could start by leaving the bank for that story, too.

Here are some common images that are used in this system, and feel free to add your own.

0 = ball, ring, or wheel
1 = paintbrush, pole, pencil, pen, straw, candle, rocket
2 = swan, duck, goose, snake
3 = heart, pair of lips, handcuffs, backside, mole hills, breasts
4 = yacht, sailboat, flag on a flag pole, table, chair
5 = s-shaped hook, cymbal and drum, seahorse, pregnant woman
6 = elephant's trunk, golf club, cherry, pipe
7 = boomerang, edge of a cliff, fishing line

8 = snowman, hourglass, egg-timer, bun, shapely woman
9 = balloon on a string, tennis racquet, tadpole, flag, monocle

You can choose one of these images or come up with your own. Then, draw your image for each image to help firmly implant it in your mind. You can use the chart below. Color in your image to make it even more memorable.

NUMBER SHAPE IMAGES		
Number	Image	Drawing of Image
0		
1		
2		
3		
4		
5		
6		
7		
8		
9		

Now take some time to reinforce this association of number and image in your mind. Close your eyes, and see each number from 0 to 9 in your mind's eye with the associated image. Make that image as vivid as possible, so you not only see the image, but you might even experience sounds, tastes, or smells associated with them, such as hearing the swan make a squawking sound. In the event you don't remember an image, look at the chart. Keep practicing until you can easily and quickly make the number and shape association.

Go through this process a few times to cement the association, and then try going backwards in reverse order. Use the chart if necessary to prompt yourself. Again, repeat this until you can do the associations quickly and easily.

Finally, come up with the numbers randomly and watch the corresponding image flash into your mind. Do this as fast as you can. Then, reverse the process, by first imagining the images in a random order and as quickly as possible connecting the number to it.

These exercises will help to solidify the link in your mind, so when you have a number to remember, you can quickly come up with the appropriate images and create a story that incorporates all these images. Once you do, visualize the whole story several times in your mind, so you encode that story with the images into your memory, and can thereafter call it up to remember the numbers by translating the images in the story into numbers.

So now start practicing. Pick out any numbers you want to remember—or generate some random number combinations—and start creating stories for the associated images, visualize them again several times, and try calling up these images to remember the numbers later to see how well you did.

Using the Number Rhyme System

As an alternative to the number shapes system, you can use rhymes instead. In the number rhyme system you use an image association for a word that rhymes with the name, instead of having the same shape, though the word you come up with might have the same shape and rhyme.

This system works exactly the same way as the number shapes system, though with rhyming images. As in the shapes system, make the associated image as dramatic and colorful as you can, so you can really see it and experience it with other senses like hearing it, feeling it, and touching it in your mind's eye. Then, using that rhyming image, you create a story linking those images together to remember the number.

The rhyming word you choose should be one that can have a clear visual image associated with it. For example, for 1, some popular associations are bun, sun, gun, and nun, which are all nouns you can clearly picture. By contrast, words like "fun" and "done" might not be good associations, since they are hard to turn into a concrete visual image.

Some possible words that are commonly used include the following:

0 = hero
1 = bun, sun, gun, nun, hun
2 = shoe, glue, pew, loo, crew, gnu
3 = tree, flea, sea, knee, bee, key
4 = door, moor, boar, paw, sore
5 = hive, chive, drive, dive
6 = sticks, bricks, wicks, licks
7 = heaven, Kevin
8 = skate, bait, gate, date, weight
9 = vine, wine, twine, line, sign, pine

As in the number shapes process above, come up with your own rhyming word or choose one from the list, and draw an image for it. Then, work on encoding that association and testing yourself as before.

NUMBER RHYME IMAGES		
Number	Image	Drawing of Image
0		
1		
2		
3		
4		
5		
6		
7		
8		
9		

Now, using the same process as before, take some time to reinforce this association of number and image in your mind. As before, close your eyes, and see each number from 0 to 9 in your mind's eye with the rhyming word and associated image. Make that image as vivid as possible, so you not only see the image, but even experience sounds, tastes, or smells associated with them, such as when you not only see the sun for the number one shining brightly, but feel the warmth of the sun shining on you. In the event you don't remember an image, look at the chart. Keep practicing until you can easily and quickly make the number and rhyme association with the particular word you have chosen.

Go through this process a few times to cement the association, and then try going backwards in reverse order. Use the chart if necessary to prompt yourself. Again, repeat this until you can do the associations quickly and easily.

Finally, come up with the numbers randomly and watch the corresponding rhyme and associated image flash into your mind. Do this as fast as you can. Then, as in learning the number shapes system, reverse the process, by first imagining the images in a random order and as quickly as possible connecting the number to it.

These exercises will help to solidify the link in your mind, so when you have a number to remember, you can then quickly come up with the appropriate images and create a story that incorporates all these images. Once you do, visualize the whole story several times in your mind, so you encode that story with the images into your memory, and can thereafter call it up to remember the numbers by translating the images in the story into numbers.

So start practicing. Pick out any numbers you want to remember—or generate some random number combinations. Then, create stories for the associated images and visualize them several times to reinforce these stories in your memory, and see how well you can later turn that story into the number you want to remember.

What's Your Number?

Now that you have had a chance to learn about and try out these different number memory systems, you can choose which one or ones are best for you under different circumstances. Certainly, you can continue to use chunking and rehearsal methods, but you may find that the methods in this chapter help to make your memory for numbers even easier by making them more vivid. And certainly it can be a lot of fun to come up with sentences, images, and stories to help you better remember your numbers.

In fact, you might find it fun to just play with numbers. For example, if you are waiting in the airport or bus station and see numbers flash in front of you, come up with a sentence or story using your associations with that number.

Or create a game to practice with others learning the system, where you race to come up with sentences or stories when you see a number. The contest can be to create the most interesting and unique story, as determined by a player who is chosen as a judge for each round; the role of judge alternates from player to player. Alternatively, take turns drawing a number and tell a story with the images associated with that number. Then, the other players race to be the first to come up with the correct number. Win a point for being the first; lose a point if you are incorrect in stating the number. And the player with the most points when the game ends wins.

Walk the Talk
Speeches, Presentations, and Meetings

Popularly, public speaking is sometimes rated as being the public's number one fear before death. At least that's what they frequently say at workshops and seminars. In any case, it is often scary, particularly when you are first starting to do this on a regular basis, and even after that, seasoned speakers and presenters, like stage actors and actresses, often feel anxious flutters before they go on. Remember, though, that having a slightly increased stress level can actually lead to a better performance, since your energy and adrenaline is up and flowing, while too much—as you may have already learned—can interfere with performance.

Perhaps the major concern, apart from people not liking your message, is that you will forget what you are going to say. When I was younger, through my 20s and early 30s, I had this fear of forgetting, though I pushed myself through it. I just forced myself to get out and speak, and eventually, after about a decade of this—practicing again and again—I got to realize that yes, hey, I can do this. I *will* remember. I *won't* forget.

Though I didn't have a particular name for the main technique I used, you might call it "tapping into your unconscious." It was like announcing I was going to talk about this particular topic, and then letting my unconscious mind loose on that subject. It's a technique I first learned at Toastmasters, when we were called upon to give a spontaneous talk for a few minutes on whatever topic the meeting leader came up with. And after I found I could do this when called on, I simply expanded the approach to other subjects, and after a time, outlines and structures for whatever I was talking about seemed to pop up into my head as well.

Well, that's just one of a number of memory strategies you can draw on to help you with speeches, presentations, and running a meeting. Here are a variety of other strategies. You've met most of them before in other chapters. The focus here is on how to apply the techniques in your memory strategies repertoire if you want to give a speech, put on a presentation, or run a meeting.

Don't Try to Memorize It All

There's no need to spend the time trying to ram exactly what you are going to say in your memory. It's a mistake to try to write and rewrite a speech or outline so you can memorize it exactly or continually repeat it over and over so you know everything line by line. While actors and actresses may have to do this in learning a part, you don't. In fact, a completely memorized talk often comes across as canned and stilted, and is likely to bore both you and your audience.[1]

Create an Outline or Mind Map with Key Words or Trigger Words

Instead of memorizing it all, focus on remembering the key words or trigger words for each topic you are going to talk about.[2] The first step is to create these words for the major topics and then create some key words or trigger words for subtopics. Then, use either a short outline of these trigger words or put them in a mind map, in which you have branches for the main topics and smaller branches coming off of those for the subtopics, as described in Chapters 11 and 17. Typically, an outline or mind map will contain up to about 100 words or less. While this approach is commonly used for speeches, you can also adapt it for presentations you are doing, such as when you are facilitating a group discussion and want to bring up certain topics. Or use this to structure a meeting and lead it with increased spontaneity and control (though you can use a written agenda as well).

Use a Visual, Peg, or Link System to Help You Remember the Trigger Word

Once you have determined your main and subtopics and the trigger words to remind you of each topic, the next step is to remember those words, and if desired, the order of those words as well. You can use any number of systems to do this. Pick the one that feels best for you. Some techniques might be:

- Create a picture in your mind of the mental map (Chapters 11 and 17); imagine you are a camera taking the picture (Chapter 23).
- Use chunking to combine subtopics together into categories (Chapter 12).
- Use the Roman Room, Loci, or other journey method, in which you put topics you want to cover along the path (Chapter 22).
- Use any of the memory techniques for recalling lists of words, such as one of the link systems and (Chapter 20).
- Use your imagination and association to make the trigger words even more memorable—as you do when you create a vivid image for each word along the path on your journey or associated with each number on your list.[3]

Decide Which System to Use to Help You Remember Your Speech or Presentation

While you can use any of these systems, sometimes you might choose one that is related to the topic of your speech or presentation. For example, if you are going to be giving a speech in a large auditorium, you might scope out the auditorium in advance and place topics at various points around the room. That way, as you gaze around the room, particular places will trigger your thoughts on that topic. Or if your talk is about gardening, you might imagine yourself walking along a path in the garden, so that certain sections of plants or objects like fountains trigger different talks. Likewise, if you are going to be giving a sales talk on cars, the journey might take you around a car showroom.

Then, whatever journey you choose, create an image for each topic that you place along the way. For instance, if your topic is increasing the bottom line for your sales talk on cars, you might see a long, white strip appear on one car you pass in the showroom; if you are going to be talking about creating a more effective phone presentation, you might see a large telephone sitting on another car.

Use Rehearsal and Repetition to Put Your Trigger Words into Long-Term Memory

Using whatever visual, peg, or link systems and imagery associations you have chosen, practice, practice, practice, so you firmly remember those words and their image associations. Then, as you call up each word on your journey or list, speak spontaneously about that topic, so you reinforce the link between the triggering words and what you are going to be talking about. You don't have to remember exactly what you are going to say; just let it flow spontaneously, which is where tapping into your unconscious comes in. Once you know the material solidly, your unconscious can take over, much like turning on a tape recorder or cassette recorder and letting it play whatever segment you select. In fact, when you let it flow spontaneously, you sound more natural and energized, which helps your speech or presentation come alive—and it makes you a better leader at a meeting too, since you are more flexible and better able to respond to whatever comes up at the meeting.

Generally, you should go through your journey at least four or five times and you should space out your rehearsals, since we learn better over time. Ideally, allow about a week to do this, and perhaps use this rehearsal schedule suggested by Dominic O'Brien, who suggests: "Play the journey over to yourself . . . at least five times; one hour after you have devised it; the next day; and then at regular intervals until the big day. According to the revision rule of five (whereby repeating something five times commits it permanently to memory), the speech should now be unforgettable, and along with it the triggers that will allow you to give a scintillating and confident talk."[4]

Using a Relaxation Technique to Overcome Anxiety

Having followed all these steps, you should now be ready. But if you still feel overly anxious—not the normal heightened level of tension that usually leads to a great performance—try a relaxation technique. Just breathe deeply and say to yourself something like "I am relaxed, I am relaxed" or "I feel very calm, cool, collected, and confident." Then, with your eyes closed or open as you prefer, imagine yourself at the start of your journey or list. Now mentally step forward or go to the first word on your list, and start talking. At this point, your unconscious should kick in and you are on your way.

Notes

Chapter 1

1. Margaret W. Matlin, *Cognition,* 6th ed. (Hoboken, NJ: John Wiley & Sons, 2005), p. 4.   2. Ibid., p. 5.   3. Ibid., pp. 5–6.   4. Ibid., p. 6.   5. Ibid., pp. 6–7.   6. Ibid., p. 7.   7. Ibid., p. 8.   8. Ibid., p. 10.   9. Ibid., pp. 10–11.   10. Ibid., p. 11.   11. Ibid., p. 99.   12. Ibid., pp. 99–100.   13. Ibid., p. 101.   14. Ibid., pp. 102–103.   15. Ibid.   16. Ibid., pp. 106–108.   17. Ibid., p. 109.   18. Ibid., pp. 109–110.   19. Ibid., p. 110.   20. Ibid., pp. 114–117.   21. Ibid., p. 112.   22. Ibid.   23. Ibid., p. 114.   24. Ibid., p. 119.   25. Ibid.   26. Ibid., p. 117.   27. Ibid.

Chapter 2

1. Matlin, p. 129.   2. Ibid.   3. Ibid.   4. Ibid.   5. Ibid., p. 131.   6. Ibid.   7. Ibid., p. 134.   8. Ibid., p. 135.   9. Ibid., p. 132.   10. Ibid., p. 135.   11. Ibid., pp. 135–136.   12. Ibid., p. 136.   13. Ibid.   14. Ibid., p. 136–137.   15. Ibid., p. 138.   16. bid., pp. 139–140.   17. Ibid., pp. 140–141.   18. Ibid., pp. 164–166.   19. Ibid., p. 140.   20. Ibid., pp. 140–141.   21. Ibid., pp. 141–142.   22. Ibid., pp. 142–143.   23. Ibid., p. 145.   24. Ibid.   25. Ibid., pp. 145–146.   26. Ibid., p. 148.   27. Ibid., p. 149.   28. Ibid., p. 150.   29. Ibid.   30. Ibid., pp. 150–151.   31. Ibid., pp. 152–153.   32. R. Sutherland and H. Hayes, "The Effect of Postevent Information on Adults' Eyewitness Reports," *Applied Cognitive Psychology,* 15 (2001): 249–263, in Matlin, p. 153.   33. Ibid., pp. 156–157.   34. Ibid., p. 506.   35. Ibid., p. 160.   36. Ibid.   37. Ibid.   38. Ibid., pp. 163–166.

Chapter 3

1. Some of these items were taken from Gary Small, *The Memory Bible: An Innovative Strategy for Keeping Your Brain Young* (New York: Hyperion, 2003), pp. 34–35.

Chapter 6

1. Karen Markowitz and Eric Jensen, *The Great Memory Book* (San Diego: The Brain Store, 1999), pp. 50, 153. Also briefly reported in David Thomas, *Improving Your Memory* (New York: DK Publishing, 2003), p. 21.   2. John B. Arden, *Improving Your Memory for Dummies* (Hoboken, NJ: John Wiley, 2002), p. 126.   3. Ibid.   4. Douglas J. Herrmann, *Super Memory: A Quick-Action Programme for Memory Improvement* (Emmaus, PA: Rodale Press, 1990) (reprinted by Blanford Press, London, 1995 and 1997), p. 40.   5. Ibid., p. 41.   6. Markowitz and Jensen, p. 102.   7. Thomas, p. 19.   8. Markowitz and Jensen, p. 102. 9. Thomas, p. 19.   10. Ibid.   11. Arden, p. 61 (similar guidelines are found in other sources, plus these are often mentioned).   12. Ibid., pp. 67–68. 13. Thomas, p. 19.   14. Arden, pp. 68–69; Markowitz and Jensen, pp. 113–115. 15. Markowitz and Jensen, pp. 111–113.   16. Douglas J. Mason and Spencer Xavier Smith, *The Memory Doctor* (Oakland, CA: New Harbinger Publications, 2005), pp. 91–93.   17. Ibid., pp. 115–116.   18. Arden, p. 73.   19. Ibid., p. 75. 20. Ibid., p. 99.   21. Ibid., p. 100.   22. Marowitz and Jensen, p. 109.   23. Ibid., pp. 122–123.   24. Ibid.   25. Mason and Smith.   26. Markowitz and Jensen, pp. 116–120.   27. Mason and Smith, p. 105–109.   28. Markowitz and Jensen, p. 120.   29. Mason and Smith, pp. 115–122.   30. Aaron P. Nelson, *The Harvard Medical School Guide to Achieving Optimal Memory* (New York: McGraw-Hill, 2005), pp. 76–79.   31. Arden, p. 101.   32. Ibid.   33. Ibid., pp. 102–103. 34. Ibid., p. 107.   35. Ibid., p. 125.   36. Nelson, p. 152.   37. Ibid.   38. Small, p. 166.   39. Max Kowrite and Jensen.   40. Ibid.

Chapter 9

1. Matlin, p. 132.   2. Ibid., p. 133.   3. Ibid., pp. 134–135.

Chapter 11

1. Matlin, p. 274.   2. Ibid., p. 275.   3. W. F. Brewer and J. C. Treyens, "Role of Schemata in Memory for Places," *Cognitive Psychology*, 13 (1981): 207–230, 1981, cited in Matlin, pp. 276–278.   4. Ibid., p. 278.   5. Ibid., p. 282. 6. Ibid., p. 283.   7. Ibid., pp. 283–284.   8. Ibid., pp. 285–286.

Chapter 12

1. Matlin, pp. 182–183.

Chapter 18

1. Matlin, p. 183; Markowitz and Jensen, p. 57.   2. Markowitz and Jensen, p. 57.   3. Ibid., p. 56.   4. Ibid., p. 57.

Chapter 19

1. Tony Buzan, *Use Your Perfect Memory*, 3rd ed. (New York: Plume, 1991), p. 69.

Chapter 21

1. Harry Lorayne and Jerry Lucas, *The Memory Book* (New York: Ballantine, 1974), p. 37. 2. Ibid., p. 38. 3. Harry Lorayne, *Harry Lorayne's Page-a-Minute Memory Book* (New York: Ballantine, 1985), p. 14. 4. Ibid., p. 23.

Chapter 22

1. Thomas, p. 38. 2. Ibid. 3. Thomas, pp. 39–40; Matlin, p. 180. 4. Matlin, p. 181 (citing a 1971 experiment by L.D. Groninger: "Mnemonic imagery and forgetting," *Psychonomic Science*, 23 (1971): 161–162. 5. Buzan, p. 65. 6. Ibid. 7. Ibid., p. 66. 8. Ibid.

Chapter 24

1. Matlin, p. 136.

Chapter 27

1. Harry Lorayne, *How to Develop a Super Power Memory* (Hollywood, FL: Frederick Fell, 2000), p. 107. 2. Herrmann, p. 199. 3. Lorayne, *How to Develop a Super Power Memory*, p. 114. 4. Dominic O'Brien, *How to Develop a Brilliant Memory Week by Week: 52 Proven Ways to Enhance Your Memory Skills* (London: Duncan Baird Publishers, 2006). p. 52. 5. Ibid., pp. 50–51. 6. Adapted from Dominic O'Brien, *Learn to Remember* (San Francisco: Chronicle Books, 2000), p. 117.

Chapter 28

1. O'Brien, *How to Develop a Brilliant Memory Week by Week*, p. 20. 2. Buzan, p. 51. 3. Ibid., pp. 51–52; O'Brien, *How to Develop a Brilliant Memory Week by Week*, p. 41. 4. O'Brien, *How to Develop a Brilliant Memory Week by Week*, p. 41.

Chapter 29

1. Buzan, p. 169. 2. Ibid. 3. O'Brien, *Learn to Remember*, pp. 104–105. 4. Ibid., p. 125; O'Brien, *How to Develop a Brilliant Memory Week by Week*, pp. 91–93.

Resources and References

Here's a list of various resources and references, many of which I consulted in the course of writing this book. If you are seeking additional information on improving your memory, these are a good starting point. In addition, you will find all sorts of memory courses and programs through an Internet search. I have included just a sampling of these.

Books

Arden, John B. *Improving Your Memory for Dummies*. Hoboken, NJ: John Wiley, 2002.

Bell, Andi. *The Memory Pack: Everything You Need to Supercharge Your Memory and Master Your Life*. London: Carlton Books, 2000.

Buzan, Tony. *Use Your Perfect Memory*, 3rd ed. New York: Plume, 1991.

Felberbaum, Frank. *The Business of Memory: Fast Track Your Career with Supercharged Brain Power*. Emmaus, PA: Rodale, 2005.

Fogler, Janet, and Lynn Stern. *Improving Your Memory: How to Remember What You're Starting to Forget*. Baltimore: The Johns Hopkins Press, 2005. (Original copyright 1988)

Frank, Stanley D. *Remember Everything You Read: The Evelyn Wood 7-Day Speed Reading and Learning Program*. New York: Avon Books, 1990.

Green, C. R. *Total Memory Workout: 8 Easy Steps to Maximum Memory Fitness*. New York: Bantam Dell, 1999.

Hagwood, Scott. *Memory Power: You Can Develop a Great Memory—America's Grand Master Shows You How*. New York: The Free Press, 2006.

Herrmann, Douglas J. *Super Memory*. Emmaus, PA: Rodale, 1990.

Higbee, Kenneth L. *Your Memory: How It Works & How to Improve It*, 2nd ed. New York: Marlow & Company, 2001. (Original edition 1977.)

Katz, Lawrence C., and Manning Rubin. *Keep Your Brain Alive: 83 Neurobic Exercises to Help Prevent Memory Loss and Increase Mental Fitness*. New York: Workman Publishing Company, 1999.

Kurland, Michael, and Richard Lupoff. *The Complete Idiot's Guide to Improving Your Memory*. New York: Alpha Books, 1999.

Lorayne, Harry. *Harry Lorayne's Page-a-Minute Memory Book*. New York: Ballantine, 1985.

———. *How to Develop a Super Power Memory*. Hollywood, FL: Frederick Fell Publishers, 2000. (Originally published in 1957.)

———. *Super Memory Super Student: How to Raise Your Grades in 30 Days*. New York: Little, Brown & Company, 1990.

Lorayne, Harry, and Jerry Lucas. *The Memory Book: The Classic Guide to Improving Your Memory at Work, at School, and at Play*. New York: Ballantine, 1974.

Markowitz, Karen, and Eric Jensen. *The Great Memory Book*. San Diego, CA: The Brain Store, 1999.

Mason, Douglas J., and Michael L. Kohn. *The Memory Workbook*. Oakland, CA: New Harbinger Publications, 2001.

Mason, Douglas J., and Spencer Xavier Smith. *The Memory Doctor*. Oakland, CA: New Harbinger Publications, 2005.

Matlin, Marget W. *Cognition*, 6th ed. Hoboken, NJ: John Wiley & Sons, 2005.

Nelson, Aaron P. *Achieving Optimal Memory*. New York: McGraw-Hill, 2005.

Noir, Michel, and Bernard Croisile. *Dental Floss for the Mind: A Complete Program for Boosting Your Brain Power*. New York: McGraw-Hill, 2005.

O'Brien, Dominic. *How to Develop a Brilliant Memory Week by Week*. London: Duncan Baird Publishers, 2005.

———. *Learn to Remember*. San Francisco: Chronicle Books, 2000.

———. *Never Forget a Name or Face*. San Francisco: Chronicle Books, 2002.

———. *The Amazing Memory Kit*. San Diego, CA: Thunder Bay Press, 2005.

Roberts, Billy. *Working Memory: Improving Your Memory for the Workplace*. London: London House, 1999.

Small, Gary. *The Memory Bible*. New York: Hyperion, 2002.

Thomas, David. *Improving Your Memory*. New York: DK Publishing, 2003.

Trudeau, Kevin. *Kevin Trudeau's Mega Memory*. New York: Harper, 1995.

Tapes and CDs

Dejong, Hans. *Silva Mind Control for Super Memory and Speed Learning*. Los Angeles: Audio Renaissance Tapes, 1994. (Original copyright 1969.)

Griswold, Bob, and Deidre Griswold. *Develop a Super Memory Auto-Matically*. Effective Learning Systems, www.efflearn.com.

O'Brien, Dominic. *Quantum Memory Power: Learn to Improve Your Memory with the World Memory Champion*. New York: Simon & Schuster, 2001.

Index

abstraction, 131
acceptance, affirming, 93–95
acronyms, 177–178
acrostics, 175–177
activities, imagining, 101–102
affirming acceptance, 93–95
aging, memory loss with, *vii*
alarms, as reminder systems,
    118–119
alcohol use, 81
all about me principle, 105–109
alphabet system, 181–186
    building image associations in,
        183–185
    choosing words for, 182–183
    game for using, 185–186
announcing technique, 160
anxiety, *see* stress
Appointments Results Forms,
    120–122
Appointments Scheduler Forms,
    120–122
Arden, John B.
    on alcohol and stress, 81
    on sleep, 70–71
Aristotle, 2
Atkinson, Richard, 4

Atkinson-Shiffrin model, 4, 5
attention, *see* paying attention
audio recorder, hearing like, 211
autobiographical memory, 27–30

Baddeley, Alan, 9, 10
Bartlett, Frederick C., 4
behaviorism, 3
body parts technique, 223–226
brain
    audio vs. language processing in,
        13
    effect of exercise on, 83
    fuel/nutrition for, 72–80
    learning consolidation in, 70
    memories in, 229
    types of thinking located in,
        11–12
    and use of self-reference ap-
        proach, 19
brain waves, 100
breath, focus on, 87
bulletin boards, reminder, 119
Buzan, Tony
    on alphabet system, 181–182
    on memory skills, 187–189
    on number shapes, 248
    on Roman Room system, 203–204

About the Author

Gini Graham Scott, Ph.D., J.D., is a nationally known writer, consultant, speaker, and seminar/workshop leader, specializing in business and work relationships and professional and personal development. She is founder and director of Changemakers and Creative Communications & Research, and has published more than forty books on diverse subjects. Her previous books on business relationships and professional development include *A Survival Guide to Managing Employees from Hell, A Survival Guide for Working with Bad Bosses, A Survival Guide for Working with Humans, Resolving Conflict,* and *Work with Me! Resolving Everyday Conflict in Your Organization.* Her books on professional and personal development include *The Empowered Mind: How to Harness the Creative Force Within You* and *Mind Power: Picture Your Way to Success.*

Gini Scott has received national media exposure for her books, including appearances on *Good Morning America!, Oprah, Geraldo at Large, Montel Williams,* CNN, and *The O'Reilly Factor.* She additionally has written a dozen screenplays, several signed to agents or optioned by producers, recently set up a film production company for low-budget films, Changemakers Productions, and has been a game designer, with more than two dozen games on the market with major game companies, including Hasbro, Pressman, and Mag-Nif. Two new games are being introduced by Briarpatch in 2007.

She has taught classes at several colleges, including California

State University, East Bay, Notre Dame de Namur University, and the Investigative Career Program in San Francisco. She received a Ph.D. in Sociology from the University of California in Berkeley, a J.D. from the University of San Francisco Law School, and M.A.s in Anthropology and in Mass Communications and Organizational, Consumer, and Audience Behavior from Cal State University, East Bay.

She is also the founder and director of PublishersAndAgents.net, which connects writers with publishers, literary agents, film producers, and film agents. The four-year-old service has served more than 800 clients, and has been written up in the *Wall Street Journal* and other publications.

For more information, you can visit her websites at www.gini grahamscott.com, which includes a video of media clips and speaking engagements, and www.giniscott.com, which features her books. Or call or write to Gini Scott at her company:

Changemakers
6114 La Salle, #358
Oakland, CA 94611
(510) 339-1625
changemakers@pacbell.net